"What if your head cracked open and poured out a mythology? Sapphire necklaces with exactly twelve stones. Russian grand-mothers who arrive mid-seizure. Blurry photographs of trees that don't want to be seen. A Viking helmet on the doorstep. In *I Believe in Everything*, Jen Dary turns a brain tumor into an antenna, a diagnosis into a dispatch. She prays to "Grandma God," weans a baby off poisoned milk, and finds that sometimes the most faithful thing you can do is believe the weird stuff. This is not just a memoir. This is a sacred transmission from the place where mystery lives, and where an entity called the Bigness shows up uninvited, sits too close, and tells you the truth whether you're ready or not."

—MATTHEW VOLLMER, author of
All of Us Together in the End

"In *I Believe in Everything*, a young mother's seismic diagnosis sets in motion a profound personal transformation. By turns witty and devastatingly serious, Dary's chronicle of a health crisis and its aftermath steadily deepens into an interrogation of that most vital of questions: what it means to live a good life."

—EMILY RUTH FORD, winner of the Royal Society
of Literature's V.S. Pritchett Prize

"*I Believe in Everything* is a mother's raw and luminous journey through brain tumor diagnosis, surgery, and recovery—navigating the bewildering and complex terrain of health crisis, mystical experiences, and motherhood. Jen Dary shows us how life's most devastating moments can crack us open to unexpected grace. A grounded story of hope for anyone who has lost it!"

—CYNTHIA LI, MD, doctor and bestselling author
of *Brave New Medicine*

"*I Believe in Everything* is a tribute to the space where the terrible and the beautiful meet, where trauma gives birth to connection, spiritual exploration, and purpose. Dary takes us on a journey through her brain tumor diagnosis and recovery that is equal parts eloquent, gritty, inspiring, and relatable."

—**LISA CONGDON**, artist and writer

"Jen Dary invites us to discover wonder, magic, and strength in situations that seem impossible, simply by showing us how it's done. Talking about brain tumors may not sound funny or uplifting, yet she tells her story with searing honesty, humility, and hope, drawing us into the surprising joy of what becomes possible when we open ourselves to all that is."

—**THE REV. LIZ TICHENOR**, author of *The Night Lake*

"An inspiring, humorous, and captivatingly honest account of one woman's journey navigating the realities of a brain tumor diagnosis, and the self-discovery that comes when one starts to ask the big questions."

—**SHANNON DUESCHER**, MSPAS, PA-C, Department of Neurosurgery, MedSTAR Georgetown University Hospital

"While reading *I Believe in Everything* by Jen Dary one word kept running through my mind: wonder. This memoir, this writer, this person, this life—it's all a wonder. This isn't just a memoir about a brain tumor and its aftermath, it's a memoir about hope, about grace, about being open to the possibility of something bigger than yourself. Dary's story is compelling and compulsive—once you start reading you won't want to stop. It's worth repeating: This book is a wonder."

—**COURTNEY LeBLANC**, author of *Her Dark Everything*

I
BELIEVE
IN
EVERYTHING

I BELIEVE IN EVERYTHING

A MEMOIR OF ILLNESS, MOTHERHOOD, AND MAGIC

JEN DARY

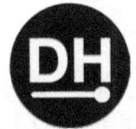

I Believe in Everything
Copyright © 2025 Jen Dary

Published by Daring House, LLC
Arlington, VA

www.daring.house

ISBN: 979-8-9990806-0-8

Cover design: Matt Roeser
Book design: Zoe Norvell
Copyeditor: Jessica Gould
Author photo: Alison DeSilva

This is a work of nonfiction. Some names and identifying details have been changed to protect the privacy of individuals.

Printed in the United States of America
10 9 8 7 6 5 4 3 2 1

To my sons: This book is for you.

AUTHOR'S NOTE

This book is a work of nonfiction. I have tried to re-create events, locales, and conversations as accurately as possible from my memories and extensive notes. I consulted with professionals to substantiate the medical information; any medical errors are my own. Some identities and locations have been changed or are composites to protect privacy. Some timelines have been condensed or expanded for readability. Thank you to my friends and family members, whose memories of the events described may be different than my own.

PROLOGUE

IT'S IMPOSSIBLE TO know what I believed in back then, before Big things arrived, when I was thirty-five years old and my sons were babies and my husband and I had never confronted *in sickness and in health*. Maybe it's simplest to say that I believed in myself and in our ability to make dreams happen. Working in tech can convince you that there's a solution for everything, that you are your only limitation, that an impressive life is always within reach.

On the morning of April 8, 2016, my sister and I went grocery shopping. Something Big was already present, but all we noticed were ambient lights and picky shoppers. Once home, I arranged my workspace and scrolled through my calendar to see who I was coaching later that day. Even now, typing this, I easily revive the ridges on my worn wooden desk, the stripes of light from skinny windows, the springy carpet beneath my feet. I felt ready for the day. And then, my phone rang. I did not recognize the number.

You know that phrase, "the first day of the rest of your life"? I'd never considered the opposite, but it's equally true: "The first day of the end of your life." That version would have sounded bleak and dramatic to me back then; I've since come to appreciate a little darkness.

But before we get to all that, before my future was both seized and protected by something Big, we have to back up a few months and start with the basics. We have to start with the headaches.

PART I

CHAPTER 1

THEY ALL TELL me I'm okay. I don't feel okay. I haven't had a day without a headache in so long.

I'm folded down in the passenger seat while Chris drives, my head near my knees. My hands cup my forehead, fingers pressing deeply into my skin.

"Find a rest stop," I whisper, the vibration of my vocal cords causing waves of pain to amplify.

We're driving home from Southern California, where I was facilitating a three-day corporate retreat for a tech company. I'm a leadership coach at Plucky, a small firm I started two years ago, and, despite the fact that Aaron is barely four months old, this opportunity was too good to pass up. The whole family came with me, my "working mother" identity on full display. I hate to ask Chris to pull over while the boys are asleep because the default is to drive-drive-drive, get as much road behind us as possible, but the pain is so bad I'm forced to do it. Within a few minutes we are pulled over at a Starbucks and I'm stumbling through the parking lot, unsure if I will need to vomit or order caffeine.

There's no line for the bathroom, a gift. I turn on the sink as cold as I can make it, running my fingers under the water, pressing them into my temple, attempting to reach the stabbing pain behind my eyes. I bow my face down toward the faucet and use my hands to pull the water closer. The distraction lifts me momentarily out of the fog.

This is really bad, I think. *I must be really dehydrated.*

Or a plethora of other things, all relatively common. Maybe I caught a virus during the retreat. Maybe three-year-old Noah brought something home from school. Maybe I have food poisoning. Whatever it is, I got it bad. I make a cold compress to go, folding and wetting three, then four grainy paper towels together.

There are still one hundred miles left in our drive, so I swallow two Advil tablets while I wait for Chris's drink order. I let the chai latte warm my hands and the red holiday cup revive my spirits. When I get back to the car, the boys are still sleeping in their side-by-side car seats. Soon we will be home.

"Better?" Chris asks as I quietly close the car door behind me.

"Kind of," I say. "Let's keep going."

———

One morning I notice the vision in my left eye is blurry. I'm taking hot, clean plates out of the dishwasher when I stand up and need to blink several times to clear the tears overwhelming my left eye. For this, I'm referred to an optometrist. Though my vision is 20/20, she prescribes me glasses with light lenses.

"Screens are stressing everyone's eyes these days," she says. "Blue light. Eye strain. You need to take it easy on the laptop."

Eye strain? For a leadership coach? I'm not looking at text all day, I'm looking at clients' faces. Plus, I just took maternity leave for three months without a single video call. Her guidance rings hollow, but because my symptoms are so nebulous, I can hardly push back. I take the prescription and choose a pair of blue wire-frame glasses. It doesn't help.

A day rarely passes without needing to pop an Advil before afternoon coaching. My clients arrive to our Zoom call, ask how I'm doing, how's the baby, how's the Berkeley spring weather? With the men, I smile, nod, and move us into the session right away. But sometimes with the women, I confide other truths.

I say that breastfeeding is easier this time, but I'm worn out and my head hurts.

"Migraines," one says. "I get one every month right before my period."

"Hormones," says another. "I had horrible headaches while breastfeeding."

We cite inspirational quotes about finding work/life balance and share podcasts about learning to say no. I allow myself to be encouraged, soothed even, by my clients. Being a woman can be mysterious, and inconvenient body issues unite us all.

But still, something is off.

I return to my general practitioner, complaining of intense muscle pain in my upper arms, then heavy stiffness in my legs, nothing consistent besides headaches, nothing obvious. I worry they think I'm a major complainer. The doctor takes me off birth control in case my hormones are causing the headaches, but it doesn't help.

For New Year's, we visit friends in Portland and I wake up in the earliest hours of 2016 with another migraine. This isn't classic migraine pain, though. I'm disoriented as I pull Chris into the guest bathroom.

"The water is too bright," I keep saying. He figures out I'm trying to talk about the light in the bathroom. I accidentally call him Dad. Later these compounding symptoms will be obvious: *Why was I not more alarmed?* But we're living the busy season of parenting very young kids who are constantly regurgitating breast milk or flinging themselves down playground slides. I'm mothering bodies newly outside my own; theirs take priority, always.

⁓

On my thirty-fifth birthday, I decide I owe it to my future self to seek different answers. Since Western medicine isn't helping, I call an acupuncturist whose office is within walking distance of our house in West Berkeley. The woman who greets me looks like Mother Nature herself, in a forest-green knit vest and brown corduroys. She smiles knowingly as I describe my symptoms, as if she already knows what the problem is, and I'm lifted by her energy. Finally, someone to help me.

I follow her down a shaded hallway into a small room, where I lay on a padded table and close my eyes. She inserts tiny needles—some in my foot, a few in my legs, a couple on my forehead—and then leaves. I lay dozing for an hour, the only sound coming from water bubbling in a fountain. It's relaxing.

On the way out, she prescribes me some herbs to mix with water and drink every day. I chug the first glass in front of her, struggling to keep my poise, but it tastes like muddy backwash. I follow these instructions for weeks, but I'm soon back to regular visits with my doctor.

One day, the doctor orders blood tests. She says the results are strange and refers me to a rheumatologist to make sure I don't have the early signs of multiple sclerosis. Navigating to another beige office building with yet another parking pass, I recount the past few months of symptoms to this new specialist. She watches me carefully as I speak.

"You don't have MS, I can tell that already. I'm more interested in why no one has done a different type of bloodwork on you. Why haven't you been referred to a neurologist?"

I rub my eyes and shift on the metal examining table. Last night, baby Aaron was awake often to nurse. I'm tired.

"Neurologist?" I say. "I don't know, this is the first I'm hearing about that idea."

I don't really want to spend time at another appointment, but I appreciate that she's asking deeper questions. Unlike any doctor so far, this one is willing to dig through the details with me. I head into the next room to be stuck with the blood-draw yet again.

The soonest appointment with the neurologist is a month away but then—serendipitously—a spot opens up the next morning. On such short notice, I have to bring Noah along, and since the nurses aren't used to having a preschooler in the office, they flood him with Post-its and stickers. Patients with canes watch us from across the room, and when I'm finally taken back to see the doctor, we've been waiting for more than an hour. I'm frustrated, but what can I say? This is the world of medicine.

Dr. Armstrong is gentle with Noah, checks my vitals and makes me walk up and down the tiled hallway, arms out. My list of symptoms includes: tired, headaches, just not feeling right. I've had migraines on and off since middle school. My sleep is interrupted many times every night to nurse my youngest. I take Advil most afternoons. Is that too much?

"Nah, don't worry about too much Advil," he says. "Take it if it relieves things. It does sound like stress. But let's do an MRI just to be sure."

Dr. Armstrong sets the expectation that it will probably take a few weeks for insurance to clear it. This is fine by me; I can't imagine what anyone would find in an MRI, and I'm heading to New York to facilitate another leadership retreat next week. I joke that I have reached my personal limit for doctor appointments in

March, anyway, and he chuckles. I make myself an easy patient.

Dr. Armstrong's report is sent through the patient portal later that afternoon, citing breastfeeding and tension as potential causes of the most recent migraines. He records that the MRI will clarify that there are otherwise no structural abnormalities. The report ends with: *Thank you for allowing us to participate in the care of Jennifer Dary, it is appreciated.*

It's a strange way to say he hopes I feel better soon.

———

"I had mono!" I laugh into the phone. "The rheumatologist sent us the report where they found Epstein-Barr antibodies in my blood. I guess I'd had mono in the fall. That must have been why I was so damn tired. Good to know I wasn't imagining all this!"

Because she's a nurse, my mom is the person you call when you're sick or when you're not sure if you can take cold medicine in addition to cough medicine in addition to headache medicine. There are apps and services these days to make you feel like you always have a doctor on call—this isn't new to me. My mom has been my personal on-call nurse for my entire life.

"Oh good!" Mom says. "When is your MRI?"

"April eighth," I say. "Early, like seven in the morning. I was thinking about canceling it because now we know about the mono, but the insurance just approved it, so maybe I should go anyway?"

Mom agrees.

It's still dark outside when the Uber arrives to take me to the radiology center. There's zero traffic, but my driver, Isaac, stops dutifully at every red light. We only have a few blocks to go when he finally speaks with a heavy accent.

"It's very early. Are you going to work?"

I use simple English to tell him that doctors need to take pictures of my head because I have headaches and that I have two young sons so we need to make sure that I'm okay. He pulls up to another red light. Then he clears his throat and tells me a story about his hometown in Peru.

A few years ago, Isaac's father was very sick. One day Isaac's grandfather (his father's father) died. At the funeral, a townswoman told Isaac's father that she knew a way for him to heal his own illness. "If someone you love dies, put a coin into their hand in the coffin and ask them to take your sickness. You will be healed," she said.

So Isaac's father did it. He placed a coin in the grandfather's dead hand, and the next day he was better. In fact, Isaac tells me, his father never needed the many medications he was taking again.

We're pulling up to the MRI office building and I'm tempted to ask questions about this creepy medical miracle. Did anyone see the coin placed in the hand? What exactly was the father's illness, and had spontaneous remission ever been studied in cases like his? Does his father seem *changed*?

But this morning I'm distracted by the impending thirty minutes in a skinny tube, so I grab my tote bag and tell him I'm very happy for his dad. He touches a strand of brown beads looped around the rearview mirror. Then, he turns around in the front seat.

"I'll pray for you," he says. "I'll pray for you and for your family."

I just have headaches, I think as I move through the dark toward the entrance. *You can save your magical prayers.*

Hours later, I will thirst for any kind of magic that exists.

CHAPTER 2

DESPITE THE EARLY hour, my sister is going to meet me in the waiting room. I tell her not to bother coming but Kate insists; when you both live across the country from the rest of your family, you graciously accept each other's help. The fact that she's a nurse doesn't hurt, either.

The woman at the desk says we'll have the results within a few days, and a technician, Anthony, shows me where to put my stuff. He says that I can wear my own clothes but have to leave my bag and shoes in a cubby. As he explains what's about to happen, I climb up on the stretcher and squeeze yellow foam earplugs until they're flat enough to slip into my ears. I close my eyes and he pushes me into the tube, then leaves the room.

"Okay, Jen," he says through the speaker, "we'll get started now. The first one will last about two minutes."

MRI machines sound like Morse code between aliens. High-pitched whines and staccato pops, as if the machine is stapling metal to aluminum siding. The stretcher shakes, too, but I keep my eyes closed and stay safely inside my own head. I figure this is the best way to avoid worrying about the ceiling collapsing in on my face.

"The next one will take three and a half minutes."

Everything's fine for the first few images, but then, suddenly,

Anthony is pulling my stretcher back out into the room.

"Something's wrong with this machine," he says. "We have to go to the one across the hall."

My earplugs are still wedged in when we arrive in the next room. Anthony tucks a new blanket tightly under my legs, retreats to his control center.

"The next one will take two and a half minutes."

But we only get through a few more images before he pulls me out again. This time, a woman in a white coat is with him. She explains that they're going to insert an IV in my arm to add "contrast." I figure this is something that Dr. Armstrong authorized, so I smile and stick out my arm.

"Have you been having headaches, sweetie?" she asks.

I nod and tell her that Dr. Armstrong ordered the MRI to make sure nothing weird was going on. I tell her I'm still nursing Aaron and ask if the contrast is dangerous for him. She agrees that I should pump and dump for the rest of the day. They push me back in the tube for the final stretch.

When they pull me out again, even more people have gathered in the room. Assuming they're residents or interns, I wave. *Did they wave back?* I don't remember. I didn't know that I would want to recall every single detail of this experience.

"Hey, thanks for talking to me the whole time," I say as Anthony shows me back toward the cubbies. "It was really helpful to know what to expect."

Anthony returns to the world behind the MRI door and I leave in the opposite direction. The woman at the front desk now says that I'll have the results within twenty-four hours. Efficient! I figure maybe it's a slow day and they bumped me up in the results queue. Later, I will understand that bumping you up is not a thing. When it's very bad, you hear right away.

I text Chris to let him know how the MRI went. *Weird, but fine,* I say. *They'll send the results later.*

Having dropped the kids at daycare, Chris is at the Reddit office in San Francisco, so our little pink house is empty when Kate drops me off. I call Mom as I unlock the front door and put my things away. She reacts a little to the contrast, though she too assumes that Dr. Armstrong ordered it as part of the scan.

Suddenly, I'm getting another call. It looks like Dr. Armstrong's number. It's 8:43am.

"Hang on, Mom, I think this is the neurologist on the other line. Let me call you back."

Thus ends The Era of Unknowing.

"Hey there, Jennifer, this is Dr. Armstrong. I'm calling because I reviewed your images and we found a large brain tumor during the MRI this morning."

Wait. What?

What?

He hasn't stopped talking, so I grab a stack of Post-its and start taking notes:

- Meningioma
- left side
- likely benign tumor in lining of the brain
- pressure on the brain
- 4-5 cm wide
- Left temporal lobe—language
- seizure discharging electrical waves
- dizzy = temporal seizures
- Seizure medication and steroid

- 3x/day Decadron
- insomnia?
- a lot of blood vessels for the work-up
- angiogram
- been around for a # of years
- swelling in adjacent main structures

None of these words make sense, but I'm not yet processing, I'm taking dictation. Coincidentally, Dr. Armstrong says, a neurosurgeon was passing his office while he was reviewing the MRI results. The neurosurgeon stopped cold when he saw the image of my tumor and asked "Who is *that?*"

Dr. Armstrong tells me: "We cannot believe you're still functioning."

It's a movie. Or a joke, maybe. Outside my window, the ignorant spring sun shines through the leaves.

He seems to be wrapping up, but I want to keep him on the phone. Maybe instinctively I know that ending this call means the beginning of something else and I want to avoid it as long as I can.

"Okay . . ." I struggle to find words. "What's your advice here?"

Dr. Armstrong pauses. "It's going to be a long road with many steps." I write these words down on the Post-it and before I can stop it, he hangs up.

—

April 8, 2016, 8:44am
To: Chris
Subject: Can you come home?
On the phone with the Dr. . . . they found something, will call you in 2 min

April 8, 2016, 9:00am
To: Friday clients
Subject: Emergency
Hi all,
If you're on this email, I have to let you know that something big has come up and I'm sorry to say I've got to move our conversations today. I'll reach out when I can, but today just ended up with an emergency I've got to handle.
Thanks for understanding,
Jen

April 8, 2016, 9:00am
Text from: Mom
Everything ok??

April 8, 2016, 9:01am
Text to: Kate
Come over when you get this, they found something

CHAPTER 3

ELEVATOR ACCIDENT. DRIVING while texting. Cancer, every cancer. Plane crashes, terrorist suitcases in the New York City subway, a mentally ill teenager with a gun at the movies. I never daydreamed about death, but if it lurked on the fringe of my consciousness, these were the more likely scenarios. A perverse part of myself is glad to finally have the answer. Oh! A brain tumor! It was out of my control.

I call Mom. Somehow I laugh as I tell her.

I laughed like this when I found out I was pregnant. I laughed like this when I was offered a job teaching English in France after graduation. I laughed like this when I was hired to fly across the country and teach Plucky workshops for the first time. It is a laughter of disbelief, one that postpones words, but up until now, that disbelief has always been about a good surprise.

Mom digs for details, so I read to her from the dictation on my Post-its. She's relieved to hear that Dr. Armstrong believes it's a meningioma. As an oncology nurse, she is terrified of glioblastomas, brain tumors that are inherently cancerous.

"A meningioma, Jen? This is *doable!*" She is really positive.

I am . . . nothing. A bystander. I'm reporting words to my mom that someone else told me and I'm not yet the patient. I'm the voice recording.

Kate comes in the front door while I'm ending the call with Mom. I don't even know if she made it home before she had to turn around. She hugs me and we talk quietly for a few minutes before Chris arrives home in tears. He crosses the room in two steps and holds me. I am numb.

"What's the neurosurgeon's name who saw the image?" Chris asks. "The one who passed Dr. Armstrong's office while it was up on the screen?"

I give him the Post-it with Dr. Taylor's information at Alta Bates.

Alta Bates Hospital is three miles away in South Berkeley. It started as a maternity hospital, named for a maternity nurse. Alta Bates is where I gave birth to Aaron eight months earlier, and it's where Kate will give birth to her daughter eight months from now. Alta Bates is a place for *babies*. It is not for *brain tumors*.

I'm still lost in this thought when I overhear Chris on the phone with Dr. Taylor's receptionist. She tells him that the neurosurgeon is booked for the next week, but Chris presses the issue and she says she'll see what she can do. Ten minutes later she's calling back. Dr. Taylor remembers the wild MRI image. Can we get there quickly? He's willing to consult with us for a few minutes before scrubbing into surgery.

Chris, Kate, and I run to the car. I check the time. The boys haven't even had morning snack at daycare yet. What. The. Fuck.

~

4/8/2016

EXAMINATION: MRI BRAIN WWO CONTRAST
Findings: There is a very large dural-based mass noted in the left anterior middle cranial fossa. The lesion has heterogeneous

T2 signal and there is significant vasogenic edema in the left temporal lobe extending into the basal ganglia and parieto-occipital region. The mass measures 5.3 x 4.3 x 4.3 cm. The lesion appears to be extra-axial with broad dural attachment and a subtle dural tail. Following contrast administration, there is homogeneous and marked enhancement of the lesion. The lesion is causing significant mass effect with compression of the left lateral ventricle. There is midline shift from left to right measuring approximately 1 cm. There are signs of uncal herniation of the left temporal lobe with impingement on the left midbrain.

The remainder of the brain appears unremarkable. No additional mass. The diffusion images are unremarkable. No findings of acute ischemia. Major intracranial flow voids are present. Left MCA branches are displaced by the mass and there appears to be neovascularity from the MCA supplying the lesion.

Released to Dr. Armstrong at Fri Apr 8, 2016 9:00am. Results have not been viewed by patient.

Brain tumor diagnosis will take hours, days to permeate. I heard what Dr. Armstrong said, but there are short periods of time when the news is secondary to the central action. I can guide Chris through traffic, I can help look for the right numbers on office doors, I can check my phone to see the time. But then—as in a violent car crash—I smash headfirst into what this news means.

We're shown back to an examination room to wait for Dr. Taylor; on the computer monitor is an image of my head, from above. I've never seen MRI film before, but the tumor is beyond obvious. Behind my left eye is an enormous white mass smashing my gray matter against the walls of my skull. A rabid invader. The image silences us all, and Chris, wise documentarian, takes a picture with his phone.

Dr. Taylor enters the office a few minutes later, all business. He explains meningiomas and assesses the figure on the screen. He sounds serious. The image looks serious. Our mood is quickly sobering.

Dr. Taylor is the first one who conveys the importance of having surgery as quickly as possible. He tells us he'd have the surgery within a week or two, tops. He suggests planning for a five-month recovery, a staggering shift to imagine in our lives. Chris takes notes:

- In left temple, between eye and ear, pushing things aside
- Is large but without lots of affect means it may have been here for years, brain has had some time to accommodate that
- Uncommon for something this big for someone this young, growing relatively quickly if you think about age
- Solid mass of pretty thick tissue
- There is some worry of it not being completely benign because you're young, it may be slightly more aggressive than a run-of-the-mill meningioma
- Very vascular tumor, there are a lot of blood vessels in this tumor, increases risk of surgery
- Surgery will be on the more difficult side. A big operation. A long stay in the hospital, long recovery
- Unclear if it's stuck to the brain or pushing on the brain
- Unknown fact: What is its behavior? Is it aggressive? Is it not?
- Out of commission for at least 3 months. Prepare

for that.

- Best thing at this point: Let everything sink in. Get ducks in a row. Be ready.

There have only been a few moments in my life when I've felt the enormity of adulthood; this is one of them. I'm thirty-five years old and my younger sister and younger husband are with me and I can't help feeling like this doctor shouldn't be telling all of this to us without our parents in the room. When I bring up the fact that I have two young sons, my voice cracks, the first tears of the whole experience, but I don't let myself go far down that path because I'm more scared than sad, more frozen than melted. It becomes clear that I need to start weaning Aaron in the next few days, as the medication prescribed isn't safe for him, and we agree that a second opinion is reasonable as a next step. We thank Dr. Taylor for squeezing us in and wish him luck on that day's surgeries.

Before we leave, I have to use the bathroom, so Chris and Kate wait for me in the office. I lock the door behind me and stare speechlessly at myself in the mirror.

How? How? How can this be real?

What about the life I thought I was going to live? Where did that go?

Do I still get a life after this? Or is this some kind of finish line?

I don't make a conscious decision to be strong in that bathroom, but I don't let my emotions overtake me either. I need to lead the two people waiting outside, and I know it will bolster them if I can convey strength. If I'm going to be out of commission, Chris and Kate need to be as strong as possible—because they're going to need to take over *everything*.

⌐⌐

April 8, 2016, 11:20am
Text from: My brother Steve
Steve: I love you so much and will be here for whatever you need,
whenever
Me: Thanks, Steve. I'm in a fog right now. I love you too xox

⌐⌐

I have built and resourced many teams. Before starting Plucky, I was the Director of Employee Development at a web agency in New York. A blend of college admissions counselor, big sister, and people strategist, I was regularly hiring and creating the best teams to do good work. But now I'm about to resource the most high-stakes project of my life: backfilling every dimension of myself.

"I'm going to grab the whiteboard," I say, heading back to our bedroom.

We will need to schedule helpers to care for our kids and household over the next few months, ask others for meals and coordinate family members to fly out. Admittedly, much of this work will be absorbed by Chris and our friends, but I'm only hours into the news and I'm not yet unhelpful.

Of course, the most important resource of all will be finding the best doctor to do the brain surgery itself. No surgeon is going to debate the fact that this giant tumor has to come out, but the surgery is risky. I want the best of the best.

Chris calls his uncle at the Mayo Clinic. Kate texts friends from nursing school and beyond. Mom reaches out to colleagues at Genentech and the various hospitals where she's worked all across the country. No one—nobody—is out of bounds. Stepping into the kitchen, I call my good friend, Leigh, whose mom runs one of the largest hospitals in New York.

"Hey friend," I say when she answers. "I need your help, it's an emergency."

Leigh is always sarcastic and witty, but she hears in my voice that I'm more serious than I've ever been. I tell her I need to find the best neurosurgeon for meningiomas.

"Okay, here's what we're going to do," she says, moving into fixer mode. "I'm going to hang up with you and call my mom. She is going to find the right person. And if it's in New York, you're going to fly here and have the surgery here. We will find people to take care of the kids."

Yes. This is a good plan. This is the solid planning I need.

"I love you, Jepting," she says, using my college nickname. "We're going to find you the best."

Within a few hours, our list stretches to the bottom edge of the whiteboard. I make appointments with several neurosurgeons in San Francisco, but by the afternoon, Dr. Michael McDermott at UCSF is the most frequent recommendation. He specializes in meningiomas, has done hundreds of brain surgeries, and is located right across the Bay Bridge. I'm lucky enough to get an appointment for the following Friday—still, it's a whole week away.

April 8, 2016, 4:41pm
Twitter
@jenniferdary: And just like that, everything is different.

CHAPTER 4

IN QUIET MOMENTS, I wonder if I somehow manifested this life-threatening diagnosis. Has my curiosity around death and ghosts and God somehow brought all this on? Maybe I've watched too many episodes of Oprah's Super Soul Sunday?

I was simply curious about the white light and the tunnel, I want to yell toward the ceiling. *I never said I wanted to go there!*

For much of her career, my mom worked as a nurse on the oncology floor, and what I remember most about her job are the stories she brought home over dinner every night.

"Today my patient said he saw Jesus in the corner."

"The same guy who was talking to his dead mother the other day? Mom, is he making that up?"

"Listen, I didn't see anything in the corner. But I believe he did."

She always said it like that. *She* didn't have an experience, but she never doubted the patient's story, either. It killed me that my mom didn't ask these patients more questions: Did the corner feel colder than the rest of the room? How did Jesus look; please include descriptions of hair, clothing, were there lambs nearby? Could the patient ask his mother what the afterlife was like, any cheat sheets for getting in?

But while Mom was very regular in reporting these stories, she also was oddly not interested in getting more details. She was a busy cancer nurse; there were always more patients to see, doctors and their egos to navigate, families to support through bad news. Take a number, Jesus. The nurses have charting to do.

Ever curious, I interviewed one of Mom's nurse colleagues for a research paper on near-death experiences in the ninth grade. Nurse Barbara told me a story about a man who was having a heart attack. Medical staff had a hard time restarting his heart using cardiac paddles, but eventually it worked. Afterward, he told Barbara that he had been hovering in the room the whole time.

"He knew details about the scrunchie I was wearing," she said. "It was nuts! How could he have known that? We have all kinds of unexplainable things happening in the hospital."

If hovering souls and Jesus lurked around hospital corners, where did that leave church? My family attended a small Lutheran church near my childhood home, an hour north of New York City. Church would have been an obvious venue to share mystical experiences, but personal stories were low on the priority list. First, we had to get through all the Bible stuff.

St. Andrew's Sunday School students learned the books of the Bible by memorizing a song. We created baseball cards for the main characters with pictures on one side, stats on the other.

Name: Sarah
Age: 127
Husband: Abraham
Fun fact: I had a baby when I was 90 years old!

Especially as I grew into a teenager, I found this dynamic lame. Memorize the facts, suppress the experience. I left for college with some historical knowledge of the Bible but nothing to help me through dating or how to negotiate a raise or choose a major, so I stopped going. Instead, I sought guidance from professors during my four years at Muhlenberg College, from formative experiences abroad, and from the kind of deep, spiritual conversations only possible after midnight, often accompanied by a few rounds of drinks.

Now, this life-threatening diagnosis is throwing me back into the God stuff.

I consider looking for my old Bible in a box in the attic, unsure what I'd do if I found it. Sing a Psalm? To cover my bases, I shoot off an emergency email to a local Berkeley psychic that comes highly recommended on Yelp. She is booked with clients for months. No dice. With repetitive words, I pray to unresponsive air: *Dear God, help. Help me. Help. Amen.*

My worst fear is that this brain tumor is cancer.

Please don't let it be cancer. Pleasepleasepleasepleasepleasepleaseplease. I can take horrible, I can work through painful, but please let it not be a surprise cancer diagnosis. I don't know if my hope can hold up against that.

I call on every dead person I know. Feisty relatives, a classmate whose cancer reoccured when we were 31, a fellow Muhlenberg student who died in a car accident one week after graduation.

Aunt Pearl, please. Use your sass, convince someone Big out there to let me stay.

Jonny. You know I wouldn't ask this unless I needed it. Please spend your cred for me. Find out who's in charge and make my pitch.

Gabe. We pondered the afterlife in the study lounge late at night. Tell me there is one. Tell me I'm not allowed in yet. I will do good with the extra time I'm granted, I swear to whatever is God.

And I do. I swear it so often that I can see it. I will be a good mom, I will find a way to coach more people, I will bring my ideas for Plucky to life. I will I will I will I will, all future tense. *Please, someone up and out there, please let me exist in future tense.*

⌒

Chris is driving, so I text my client on the way to pick up the kids.

Hey—need to talk for a minute when you can. (Emergency)

We're rounding the corner of San Pablo when Mark calls.

"I have some big news," I say. "I had an MRI this morning and we found a big brain tumor so I have to close Plucky for a while."

"Oh my God. Fuck."

We're paused at a crosswalk to let a woman in a sari cross with two kids. One of them is skipping.

"We're going to get a second opinion," I say. "I mean, it's clear I need brain surgery, but we don't know when yet."

"This is fucking garbage. Oh my God. Jen, what do you need?"

No. I'm *his* coach. I'm the one who asks *him* this question. I help *him* process challenges and big changes.

"Thanks, we're going to pick up the kids now. I don't need anything. We're trying to figure this out."

I can't stop speaking in short sentences. I'm so awkward.

"Whatever you need, Jen, call. We will send anything. We will jump on flights to be there."

It's outrageous, what he's offering.

"Yeah, thanks. Really, thanks. I'll keep you in the loop about next steps."

Keep you in the loop? Next steps? I don't have language for any of this without making it sound like a business transaction. Chris parks our old gray Honda Civic in front of Bright Horizons daycare.

Don't look at me, I think as we pass the always-friendly woman at the front desk. *Don't ask me how I am, how my day is going. I have no idea what to tell you.*

We stop in Noah's class first and collect his things: dinosaur lunchbox, blue backpack, sports-themed water bottle, green

Oakland A's cap, and a piece of recently dried artwork. He runs ahead to Aaron's classroom and peers through the long skinny window of the infant room to find his brother. Aaron's teacher waves us in and we are tight, quiet, tense. Maybe the teacher thinks we had a fight on the way over or that we're very tired after a long week. What reason would there be to think otherwise?

The names of these pills, I've forgotten, but Dr. Armstrong is adamant that I start them right away. One pill will cause insomnia. One pill will make me tired and sluggish. Starting now, I'm not allowed to drive.

After these drugs hit my system, my milk will be unsafe for Aaron, so Chris is researching formula options from the couch. Frozen milk will tide us through a few days and then my boy will be moved to formula. *This was not the plan!* The temptation to be angry surges, but it feels like my house is burning down and I can only save what I can carry. Emotions are too heavy, so I leave them behind and focus on the physical, the tangible. I place the first of four pills on my tongue and sip water to push it down. Now, for my body, this is all real.

Once the boys are tucked in, I sit on the edge of my bed and call my other clients, one after the other. Every time it's the same. Clients are stunned and uneasy. They make declarations about my fortitude and vow to do whatever I need.

What will happen to Plucky if I die or am impaired by brain surgery? Plucky is a pile of ideas, a good website and a doable part-time income, but so far that's about it. My coaching clients will find new coaches. My consulting clients will find new consultants. I'll be easy to replace.

CHAPTER 5

THE NEXT MORNING, Aaron's babbling draws me out of
sleep. Our room is dark and the fan is blowing. I snuggle down
under the electric blanket, resisting the morning.

BRAIN TUMOR. Now I'm awake, remembering. *BRAIN
TUMOR.* Today is Saturday. Yesterday was the worst day. *BRAIN
TUMOR.*

Chris gets up, closes the door softly behind him. I hear him
pouring Noah a cup of milk and defrosting breast milk to make
Aaron his bottle. Their voices are muted through the bedroom door,
but not by much. I check my phone, see a text from Mom.

*Good morning, my daughter! I hope you got some sleep last night!
Call me anytime, we love you so much!*

I stop by the bathroom on the way to the living room. Same
chin-length, wavy hair. Same mole on my left cheek. I lean my
face closer to the mirror, looking for secret information behind my
left eye. This blue eye never told me there was a lemon-size tumor
pushing against it. Traitor.

"Mommy!" Noah cheers and crawls onto my lap. Aaron smiles
from where he has pulled himself up on the couch. He drops to the
floor and speed-crawls over to me.

"Hello, my babies," I say, kissing them both on their soft hair.

"How did you sleep?"

Chris sets up *Octonauts* while I pour my coffee. Champion.

We met at work. Having recently completed a Master's degree in Paris, I returned to New York just in time for the 2008 financial crisis. Despite having only basic technical skills, I was hired at a web development agency to write copy for an app that a young, superstar developer built in a single weekend. Chris Dary was a well-liked, hard-working developer from Wisconsin. I liked him a lot, but I was also trying to avoid getting fired, so I decided I would never date him. Eight months later, I'd failed and fallen swiftly in love.

We were married at an arboretum near my parents' house in New York. We worked with the pastor to write our wedding ceremony, using very simple language, opting out of the religious and prioritizing what sounded authentic. That said, we did keep a few traditional elements, vowing to stick together in sickness or in health.

Now we've been spouses for four years, parents for three. The intense transition to parenting allied us on the same team; Chris plus Jen equals parents, plural. This brain tumor news shoves us into very separate categories: one healthy parent and one who might die. I'm already distancing myself.

"What should we do today?" I can tell my husband is trying to keep things light as we both monitor my mood. Our plan had been an Ikea trip to find a small dresser for socks and diapers, but visiting an enormous Swedish warehouse seems sacrilege. That said, I'm failing to imagine which activity would be more appropriate. *BRAIN TUMOR.* What *do* you do? Drape the mirrors and weep with fear? Our sons' needs override any poetic ideas I can come up with.

"I mean, what if we still went to Ikea?"

Chris laughs. "I'm okay with that if you are."

"Let's do it," I say. "I'm going to jump in the shower."

I'm halfway down the hallway when Chris yells to me. "Did you take your meds yet?"

Ah. I turn back toward the kitchen, collect the pills, and swallow them down. A new routine begins.

———

Published on PERSONAL BLOG
April 9, 2016
8:28pm

Title: So.

I have a brain tumor.

There's no other way to start this. I've written and rewritten this a hundred times but here's where we are. Yesterday morning I had an MRI to make sure that my last six months have been full of tension headaches and nothing weird. My sister waited in the waiting room while I went into the tube where they took pictures of my brain. Then ten minutes after I got home, the neurologist called and said they found something.

I called Chris and told him to jump in an Uber. I called my sister and asked the same thing. Soon they were here in the living room and we were on the phone with the neurosurgeon. Then we went to his office. It was crazy news! How insane! And that's how I felt until I saw this image when we walked into his office and I saw the motherfucking large tumor behind my left eye. And then I felt very scared.

There is no way to write this post well.

I'm not interested in:

Dying. (Please. I have a whole lot of things to do on the planet for humans.)

Losing abilities to speak or walk or parent or function.

Losing the ability to speak French (DO YOU KNOW HOW MANY DOLLARS I SPENT learning French. Do you know how long I lived there? I adore this language and the people there. Let's get this tumor out of the left temporal lobe because that's where it is affecting my language.)

I'm also not interested in someone cutting open my skull, existing in ICU for a while, closing down Plucky for months while I recover, missing planning and hosting my baby's 1st birthday party . . . but I guess you have to choose your battles.

So. Yesterday was the worst day of my life. And I'm not looking forward to a lot of the next few months, but here we are. The outlook looks good, but I have a meningioma in my left temporal lobe and it's soon time for brain surgery. We've got some things to talk about.

xo

⌒

In all, 256 people comment on Facebook when I share this blog post. They emerge from all parts of my life—elementary school to grad school, friends in other countries, former coworkers, my friends' parents and my parents' friends, people who were cooler than me and people who are cooler than me, still. As they react to each other's comments, strangers liking strangers' words in an effort to build my confidence, they're telling a story that I'm not sure I believe.

Jen, this tumor has nothing on you.

Jen, you're a warrior.

Jen, you will be back in action before you know it . . . watch out, world!

I lay awake for most of the night, their profile pictures swimming in front of me. Around 2am, I realize I need a strategy for calming my mind and I remember the practice of Metta. I heard about it once on a podcast. In this meditation, you identify a person and hope three things: that they are well, that they are safe, and that their life unfolds with ease. But before you get to other people, first you have to start with yourself.

May I be well. I try to picture what well would feel like. I imagine *feeling* well, like I'm untouchable by such difficult news because the true question of wellness lives in a peaceful place, deep inside of me.

I am proud of who I am. I'm kind and I'm funny. I have a family (and 256 commenting people) who love and support me. My chest feels full, my shoulders strong, and my heart warm. Despite the past two days, I *do* feel well with myself.

Next, I move on to safety.

May I feel safe. Unlike wellness, safety is more circumstantial. When I visualize the MRI image, I feel unsafe. That foreign, large mass behind my eye is invasive, and the unknown feels extremely dangerous right now.

Instead of the tumor, I focus on the doctors who have studied hard to learn how to carve tumors carefully away from a person's living, necessary brain. I appreciate Anthony, the MRI technician, and Dr. Taylor's receptionist, who got us in to see him between appointments. These people are helping to make a dangerous situation safer for me. I breathe in and out and feel their efforts as a net underneath me. I feel safer.

Now for the hard one.

May my life unfold with ease. Un-fold-with-ease. Good, meaty words.

This brain tumor is an enormous reminder that I can't control everything. The last time I let things physically unfold was during natural births with both my boys, when one of the biggest things I learned in labor was to not work *against* my body. If I was scared, my muscles would tighten and this would tire me out. I had to actively practice letting my body do what it needed to and not get in my own way. *What would it look like to work with the tumor, not against it?*

In this way, the experience before me opens as a potential curriculum. I feel myself simultaneously coach and client, guiding myself and processing myself and it's—well? Trippy.

Still wide awake, I do Metta prayers for friends and family, remembering how we met and wishing them well. In almost every case, I'm awed by how many circumstances conspired to bring us to each other's lives. The math of the universe is overwhelming, and not one aspect of my life seems random or accidental. I decide to believe that my brain tumor has been written in the stars, as if it was my choice originally. When I feel untethered, I come back to this safe mental island, where I've chosen a daunting path for a reason.

What if this is the story that I've been training for?

It's the safest perspective that I've found so far. I drift off to sleep.

～

I know someone you need to talk to, Wil texts. My client connects me with his friend in Seattle who had a brain tumor several years ago. I'm eating a donut on the front steps when she calls. (Who would eat a salad for lunch when their life's on the line? Truly.) Geraldine is funny and calm.

"It's worse than you think it will be," she says. "But it's also better." I confirm that people have been amazing so far.

Geraldine talks about post-op times when her Italian switched with English. Also how tired she was, how much she slept. It's helpful to talk to someone in the brain tumor club, but during this phone call, I realize that our clubhouse is diverse. Geraldine's tumor was benign and hopefully mine is too, but our tumors are in different areas of the brain, so our long-term side effects will affect different neuro-motor functions. After we hang up, I stay in the sun a while longer, imagining how things could have been if the diagnosis had come at a different time. What if we were still in New York? What if we weren't yet married? What if it was before Plucky or before kids or even after our kids were grown? All of these potential lives have different shapes, some more tragic than others.

Most of what I'm anxious about is recovery with kids. How will it ever be possible to do all of the necessary sleeping Geraldine describes? We live in a small two-bedroom house. The living room and hallways are death traps of small cars and trains and loud, light-up electronic toys. There isn't room for peace and quiet—which means that there will be an even heavier burden for Chris and my family to keep the kids calm or out of our tiny condo. I hate what I must ask of them. *I'm* the capable one, the flexible one, the one who takes a problem and runs with it.

Geraldine's simplest guidance is to go slow and have hope. I'll try.

―

A small box, addressed to me, arrives with the mail. Inside is a metal stand and a circular piece of cushioned fabric, like a yarmulke for some giant's head. There's no note, but the packing slip lists my friend Greg as the sender. The boys take turns balancing the giant yarmulke on their heads and we take pictures, which I text to Greg.

Me: Is this from you?

Greg: There should be another box too. Then it will make sense. Just you wait . . .

Two hours later, another box arrives. First, I see fur. Packing Styrofoam bits fly onto the floor as I lift out an enormous helmet. Horns and all, it's heavy. Noah cheers.

"What is it, Mom? What is this?" I look across the room at Chris, who answers for me.

"It's a helmet! A Viking helmet!"

"Oh man," I say to Chris. "You have to take my picture."

I lift the beastly helmet onto my head. It's unwieldy but funny, and my stomach is a mix of joy and embarrassment. How much did Greg spend on this? He didn't have to; he's a busy guy. I upload the helmet picture to my Facebook profile and publicly thank Greg for the gift. Hundreds of friends chime in, and a college classmate surprises me with her comment.

Thank you for allowing your FB family to share in your life, she writes. *I hope that you pour out some of your fears and let us bring some light and laughter into yours. Rock on, lady!*

I'm not the only one waiting to see how this story ends. The war will be mine alone, but my community is arming me for the fight.

If you google "ways to relieve engorgement," you find cabbage leaves right at the top of the search results. Engorgement happens a few days postpartum when your milk is first coming in, before your body knows how much milk your baby needs. Engorgement can also happen when you wean your baby—especially if you're trying to stop quickly, from one day to the next. I'm feeling real cool today, walking around with a brain tumor and old cabbage leaves in my bra. At least it's a distraction.

This is all so ironic because breastfeeding didn't come easy to me. Before Noah was born, I read a few books and took a breastfeeding class, but I thought my body would automatically know what to do. I put him to my breast and assumed he was eating, but every time we went back to the pediatrician, Noah was lighter and lighter. Then, when he was a few days old, we found crystals in his diaper.

The pediatrician did not mess around.

"Will you bring me some formula?" she called to the nurse down the hall.

Noah was dehydrated. I had no idea. We hired a lactation consultant that afternoon, and it took her guidance and a breastfeeding support group to get my body to work with Noah's, but eventually it did work.

This time around, working from home has made nursing and pumping easier. It's been my plan to wean Aaron around his first birthday, but that's three months away. With the introduction of Keppra and Decadron, there will be no poetic nighttime-only feedings, no time for sentimentality. Unknowingly, I've already nursed my son for the last time.

Aaron sits sleepily on the floor in his sleep sack, just up from his nap. Chris has brought home a few different formula options and mixes one at the sink. When the bottle's ready, I measure out my afternoon dose of meds and slip a fresh cabbage leaf in each side of my bra.

"I can't be here," I say. "I think he'll do better if he takes it from you." I shuffle back to the bedroom, where I lie down, large chunks of my mother identity spinning away.

Later, it will be hard to feel his desire to nurse and need to refuse him. I will have nightmares about a popular cheerleader from high school nursing him, stepping in because I can't. *A mother is not everything*, I think. Others can feed my baby, others can protect him. I'm downplaying my value, unwinding my role because it hurts too much to stay close and imagine what may come anyway.

Chris calls back to the bedroom a few minutes later. "He sucked it all down!"

Thatta boy, I think, but I'm too tired to call back.

CHAPTER 6

THE FIRST CRANE to arrive is from my friend Sean. Inside the envelope is a wadded-up piece of pink construction paper. *This looks more like a dinosaur than a crane,* he writes. *Jess told me about everything and I had to try. I'm thinking of you from Philly!* Who would craft an origami project when a small card would have been so much easier? But then Chris brings the mail in and there are two more cranes in envelopes. These cranes actually look like cranes.

We track down the origin story. Lindsay, a fellow Muhlenberg grad, has alerted dozens of friends, going beyond just the freshmen ladies of third floor Prosser Hall. Cranes are arriving from Lindsay's local friends in Durham, folks who have never met me, from my aunt and uncle in Pennsylvania, from my mom's coworkers at Genentech. I'm embarrassed to think that people have spent time learning how to fold a paper crane. At the same time I realize that I was afraid there would be a few cards, flowers, nothing more. It matters to me if I'm remembered.

Another friend teaches her entire fifth-grade class how to make cranes. They arrive in a box, 27 imperfect cranes made by children, and when these cranes arrive, my embarrassment gives way to something else. I imagine their small fingers folding paper because their teacher told them a story about me, and I feel her leadership, her intention. I admire her ability to amplify her love and suddenly I stop feeling embarrassed. Instead, I start to feel prayers.

With every fold of paper, stamp stuck on an envelope, handwritten mark of a pen or stroke of a key, a human being is offering me their loving energy. I'm bolstered by it—in fact, I can't sleep because of it. Besides insomnia, I lay awake all night remembering and marveling at and loving the people behind every generous gesture that came in that day.

⌒

Chris shuts the door to the boys' room. I hear him turning off the lights in the living room, now the kitchen, then he pokes his head around our bedroom door.

"I'm going to brush my teeth and get into bed," he says. "Need anything?"

"No," I say softly. "Just resting."

I hear the sink turn on in the bathroom and look at the clock. It's 7:15pm.

"How are you?" he asks as he slides into bed next to me. We're facing each other, heads on pillows. The cats are asleep at the foot of the bed.

"I'm okay," I say. "I just can't ever fall asleep. I'm like a zombie. Maybe I slept three hours in the past day."

"Well, there's nothing to do tonight. I'll get the boys if they wake up. You can just relax and try to sleep."

"Thanks, love, I know." I make a face.

"What's that face?"

"I feel like we should talk about some stuff, but there's never a good time when the kids aren't here and we're not exhausted."

"Let's talk about it," Chris says. "I'm going to leave my head on this pillow, though."

"I don't really want to get into this, because we know I'm going to be fine and my odds are good and probably McDermott will be my surgeon. But I just want to tell you that if something happens, I want the boys to have a mom."

Chris nods. He takes my hand. We talked about this before tumors; in early parenthood we gave each other permission to find new partners if something ever happened to the other.

"I mean, we would probably move back to New York to be near your parents," Chris says. "Or I guess now that Kate is out here, I don't know . . ."

"We don't need a plan," I say. "But I want you to know I still feel strongly about that, and any decision you would make would be totally good by me."

In the movie version, we would cry, but we're both so exhausted that we flirt with and avoid the conversation about dying. We lay like this for a while, still holding hands. At some point Chris falls asleep and I look over his face in the soft lamplight, watch him breathe in and out. The beauty of the moment is unbearable, so I roll over and turn out the light.

The underground parking lot at UCSF Parnassus is so full that we have to keep making tight turns to descend to lower and lower levels. It's sobering to see how many people are here today and to realize how many days in my life I *haven't* had to be at the hospital. I've been lucky.

The University of California San Francisco Medical Center is made up of three hospitals. We're meeting Dr. McDermott at UCSF

Parnassus, a six-block chunk of buildings clustered on a hill over-looking Golden Gate Park. From its earliest days, UCSF has been an excellent teaching hospital, and, besides doing brain surgeries, Dr. McDermott mentors young neurosurgeons there, too. Walking around Parnassus even feels like visiting a university: Admissions, the cafeteria, a campus map that we check to make sure we're on the right side of the street. When an ambulance passes, sirens trumpeting, we're reminded that we're not at college. At Parnassus, we're deep in emergency territory.

Starbucks is half a block away and filled with doctors and nurses, students and people like us. As we wait to order, I'm feeling unprepared to meet Dr. McDermott. I don't have questions or an outline, and I'm mostly relying on my gut and the recommendations of those I respect. More than a dozen people endorsed him in our search to find the best meningioma neurosurgeon in the country. In my mind he's a king, a slayer of brain dragons, master of cutting you open and extracting only the parts that don't belong, leaving you—your personality, your functions, your memories—intact.

Through Plucky coaching, I've observed that people do their best work when they care about their job and believe that their efforts matter. I want the person who opens my head to feel appreciated and motivated to do good work. It's in my best interest that Dr. McDermott love his job when he does my brain surgery—if he will have me. So I ask the barista for some advice.

"Hey! So, uh, weird question? I'm meeting with a neurosurgeon in a few minutes about removing my brain tumor and I'd like to bring him something to say thanks. What would you recommend?"

She's taken aback . . . but not that much. This is a barista on a hospital campus, and I feel sure that she's been involved in many emotional pastry orders before today. Still, she holds my question at arm's length, staying outside the details.

"Wow, uh, I don't know. A slice of lemon loaf?"

"Great. Lemon loaf it is!" I announce. Chris shakes his head as we move toward the register to pay. I write a few words on the Starbucks bag, a pre-thank you note, while Chris gets his coffee. Now I feel more ready, more myself, with gift in hand. We find our building and head to the elevator. Once inside, a woman close to the buttons asks where we're headed.

"Eight, please," Chris says.

I wonder if the others in our crowded elevator know that we're headed to the brain tumor floor, if they imagine it's because of me or Chris or if it's one of our parents or grandparents. I face a framed poster about upcoming events at UCSF and catch my reflection in the glass. Man, do I look tired.

"What time is your appointment, one fifteen?" Chris murmurs, and I nod. A man in scrubs glances in my direction. *There's the big reveal,* I think. *It's me. I'm the tragedy today.*

What strikes you first about the Department of Brain Tumors is the view from the waiting room. Overlooking green parks, some fog, and, farther back, the Golden Gate Bridge, it's the money shot. A few patients are also waiting for appointments, many shepherded by a friend or family member. Some are bald. A few use walkers or canes. Not everyone is old.

Chris checks me in at the front desk because the short walk to and from Starbucks has taken all my energy and I'm crashing. I sit facing away from the spectacular view and try to recharge. When we're called back into the office, a nurse practitioner takes down some notes and tells us Dr. McDermott will be in shortly. He's late, but not that late, and when he enters the room and shakes our hands, it feels like meeting a celebrity.

Dr. Michael McDermott has small, circular glasses that make him look smart. He isn't memorably tall but he holds himself with formality. He speaks calmly, not too loud or hard to hear. He's Canadian, originally from Toronto. I tell him about some Plucky travel I've done to Toronto, and he smiles when I make a joke about the names of Canadian coins—loonies and toonies. After introductions, he reaches for a small penlight in his breast pocket and rolls his stool over to me. He tells me to look straight ahead.

"I see you have papilledema."

"What's papilledema?"

"Swelling because of elevated pressure that's been present for some time." He rolls on his stool to look into my other eye. "Okay, more on this side, a big one there."

"Are those going to cause permanent damage?" Chris asks.

"Those are from high pressure. The headaches are a manifestation of elevated intracranial pressure."

That I do not understand all of what he's saying makes me trust him more. Dr. McDermott rolls over to the desk where the MRI image of my brain is displayed on a monitor.

"So this is a meningioma, a tumor that arises outside of the brain's substance. It rises from the covering of the brain, called the dura. There's some boney change here." He gestures towards the screen. "See the big white shadow here? Your brain shifted over; it's twisted way over to the other side, but you're walking and talking and doing fine."

He's right. My brain has been accommodating to the intruder.

"Look at the vessels coming out of here, these linear streaks," he says. "These are all blood vessels coming from the artery. It's kind of pretty, no?"

A man who loves his work. My heart thuds. This is exactly how I need McDermott to be.

"As terrified as I am, this is super fascinating as a human," Chris jumps in, and the whole situation is bizarre, as if we are listening to a live RadioLab podcast. He's not wrong; it is interesting, but for the fact that this brain tumor is inside my own head.

"It all depends what you do, right? For me it's just another day at the office. . . ." Dr. McDermott trails off.

"How long do you think I've had this?"

"Years."

"And do you think it grew larger from hormones from my pregnancies?"

"Maybe."

Chris jumps in. "Do you think it's cancer?"

"No. The big ones most often tend to get called grade 2, but when we take them out, they frequently do not come back. It's probably better to get this done sooner rather than later because your brain has shifted a lot. We could push to get it done next Thursday, but I think we're fine to wait for the following Monday."

Seven days ago I was naive to everything. Now an emergency brain surgery will be happening in ten days and it will be happening to me.

"It's the craziest thing," I say. "They kept telling me I had two young kids and a business and that's why I was stressed."

"No one looked in your eyes?" And with this one question, the entire American medical complex falls to pieces.

Did anyone look in my eyes? No. Or if they did, they saw what they wanted to see. In a way I can hardly blame them; a thirty-five-year-old mom to young kids who runs a business *is* stressed. But I was following something larger than logic, a scent or an instinct that would not relent until I found someone who'd simply look into my eyes. Dr. Michael McDermott has earned his lemon loaf.

"The risk profile with this kind of surgery is within an acceptable range, but I need to stress it's not none," he continues. "We're probably going to shave your hair back and put the skin incision all the way across and fold your skin down. Because the tumor goes along the floor of the skull, we'll do an orbito-zygomatic craniotomy through a left frontotemporal approach. We have to get out the bone and I have to get to the floor, so I'm going to make a cut in this arch"—he points to my eye area on the screen—"and drill down that bone so I can get to the floor to get out all the tumor and its attachments."

I've basically stopped listening, because it's all too weird and gross and real. I'm worried about death from so many angles that the risk of dying during brain surgery is just one more added to the pile. Also I don't need to pay close attention, since Chris is recording and taking furious notes.

"Is there a chance her language will be affected?"

They go back and forth about how temporary or permanent my language damage could be. Chris tells a story of how I slumped over the other night at dinner; Dr. McDermott confirms that I'd had a seizure. Chris asks about the rate of stroke. I sit back and let them do this together, Chris mastering medical terms for all of the invisible moments he's been observing.

"How many of these surgeries have you done?"

Dr. McDermott doesn't miss a beat. "About 1,200."

I wonder if I can just sleep in his office until the surgery, listening to him read people's MRIs all day, dozing to the sounds of his plans for attachments and arteries.

"Let's talk post-surgery," I say. "Dr. Taylor said that I'd be in the hospital a week, and then three months recovery. Does that sound accurate?"

Dr. McDermott cringes. "I hope not." We all laugh. "Two months recovery, maybe," he adds quietly.

The whole appointment lasts less than an hour. I thank him several times and offer him free leadership coaching for life. These kinds of sentences fly off my tongue at this point, a full-fledged resistance to leaving planet earth. I can't imagine coming to these appointments without some aspect of begging for your life. His hand is on the doorknob, but he turns before he leaves.

"I'll do a good job," he says, meeting my eyes. "You can trust me."

CHAPTER 7

I HAVEN'T BEEN alone in public in over a week and I want
to take a walk. I throw a sweatshirt on top of my pajamas and slide
into my bright red Toms.

"I'm going to 4th Street," I tell Chris. "I need to do something
normal."

We live in a little historic area of West Berkeley, just a tenth of
a mile from the shop-lined, active 4th Street. The houses on our
block are painted charming colors like pale blue and dusty pink.
They look old, but, with a few exceptions, they were mostly built in
the 1980s. Chris found our tiny two-bedroom house when he flew
out for Reddit onboarding, and it wasn't until Noah and I officially
arrived that I saw it in person. In the months since we brought
Aaron home, we've been talking about a bigger space for our growing family. This idea is now off the table, for obvious reasons.

As I walk down our front stairs, freedom pulses in my chest. Oh,
how I've needed this independence! I pause to wave up at the boys
when I reach the front gate. Chris's watchful stance is clear through
the window, too, and I wave again. "All good!" I say and start walking down the wooden walkway. But I've only moved about twenty
feet when I realize I'm *not* all good. There are two streets to cross in
order to get to my destination, and I can only cross the first before

I must sit down on the curb and rest. I'm winded.

The spot of sun on the pavement in front of me is not big enough to warm my entire body, so I let it shine on my left foot. I look at the skin of my ankle, rub it with my fingers.

"Hi, skin," I murmur. "Hi, foot. You're okay."

A trail of ants is headed toward someone's dropped pastry. I watch them for a while, ants doing teamwork, efficient and driven. Maybe I'll buy a scrapbook in the stationery store on 4th Street, somewhere to keep all of the cards and letters I've received. Maybe the kids will want to read it one day, especially if . . . ?

I distract myself by taking a picture of my tired legs to post on Instagram. *Who will read these posts?* I'm awkward, self-conscious of the fine line between attention-seeking and pursuing community. Maybe it's okay to post things like this when you're really sick. Especially if . . . ?

Well. No one tells dead people they were too much on social media.

I've been sitting so long that the sun spot has moved off the sidewalk. I won't make it another block today, so I tuck my feet under me, push myself to standing, and return home.

———

"I think you're really going to do something big," he says.

Pitter patter, says my heart. My first boyfriend is flirting with me, but there's something else behind his words.

"Something big?" I laugh. "Like what?"

"I don't know." He shrugs and takes another big bite of cereal. We're upstairs in the computer room at his house. He looks up at me, conviction in his eyes. "But I would take that bet. You're going to be someone."

I dare it to be true. Teenagers take flight in such quick succession—driving and dating and college and travels. The older people in my life grumble about how this will all fall away, that my desire to see potential in the world will be squashed by bills and reality. Maybe so, but I'm seventeen and swept up in the optimism of youth, of new freedoms granted each year of my life.

Later I will see that two things were present in my first love:

First, I was in love with him, enamored with the first opportunity to hear someone else's most intimate thoughts. And to share mine.

Second, I was on fire with the prophecy he was declaring for me. *I am going to do something big. I am actually going to be someone.*

Years later, I observe that the light dies out in my relationships when my lovers grow up, when their hopes and ideas are neutered. For a while in my twenties I wonder if the truth of love is that it's a thread that appears in different people. What if the men I'm dating are vehicles for this feeling? Is my truest love not a person, but a feeling of vast potential, an awareness of all that exists, conveyed through human form?

I want to see my optimism validated, stubborn in the desire to live beyond the boundaries of my physical body. If you're lucky enough to have someone tell you that you're going to do something big, you spend your whole life looking for a way to prove it; you spend your whole life in this becoming.

Noah comes into our room and gets into bed with me.

"Hey buddy, I'm sorry I'm not playing. I don't feel so good."

"When you're sick, your family can help."

"What a smart boy you are. You and Dad and Aary *are* my helpers."

He snuggles against my shoulder. How do I tell my three-year-old what's about to happen to me?

"You know, when I see my doctor next week, he's probably going to give me a little haircut."

"Why?"

"Because he wants to make sure my head is good and I'm feeling healthy. So when I come home from the doctor, my hair might be shorter than yours!"

"Yeah!"

"What do you think, should I look for a special hat?"

"Maybe."

"What kind of hat should I wear?"

"You can wear an A's hat like me."

"Oh, that's a great idea. Then we can match."

"Two A's."

"Two A's."

—

After ten days of slowing to a halt, assignments are being given out, action picking up. My mom arrives and sets up camp in our living room, and I finally release my guilt for leaving Chris to care for the boys alone.

"Look at this!" Mom says, unzipping a large tote bag full of word puzzles and Sudoku books. "You'll be all ready to retrain your brain!"

At the moment, I'm too tired to even pick up a book, but it feels good to have someone actively planning for my recovery.

Chris rents a second car for the month so that our visitors can help with appointments and kids and groceries. Later today, a sofa bed will be delivered for our guests. When does it arrive? What color is it? I'm no longer in the know. As we approach the bridge between Before and After, I allow myself to be taskless.

―

A lady from UCSF is on the phone with instructions about my "upcoming surgery, scheduled for Monday, April twenty-fifth, two thousand sixteen."

"You'll need to check in at 10:50am. The surgery will start at 12:50pm."

I don't need to ask how long surgery will be; Dr. McDermott has already told us. It could last six hours.

"This is sounding like a long day!" I reply. "Should I bring snacks for the doctors?"

UCSF lady laughs and says no, they're actually not allowed to eat snacks while doing brain surgery, which I guess makes sense.

"What about the embolization procedure on Friday? Is there anything I need to know about that?"

UCSF lady checks my file. "No, you should be all set. Tomorrow's appointments will get you ready for both the embolization and the craniotomy."

"Okay, thanks for checking," I say. "No offense, but I hope we never have to talk again."

"Good luck, sweetie."

I accept her luck.

―

I don't know the French words for *brain tumor* or *craniotomy* or *embolization* or even *blood work*. Luckily, the admissions aide, who is taking my vitals, lets me drop English equivalents into our conversation. When I appeared at his station a few minutes ago, I found out that he's originally from Togo, a Francophone country. Coincidentally, Kate did Peace Corps in Togo, so we have things in common.

"*Ils vont me faire un* embolization," I say. "*C'est un truc où ils vont* feed a coil through an artery in my groin *qui va arrêter le sang qui nourrit la tumeur.*"

The technician is wrapping a blood pressure cuff around my arm and doesn't miss a beat.

"*Oh la!*" he says. "*Vous en avez eu des migraines?*"

I wave my hand. "*Beh, oui et non. Aussi des problèmes de la vision, aussi du stress, ce n'était vraiment pas évident ce qui se passait. . . .*"

When we emerge a few minutes later, Kate is excited to hear about the Togo connection.

"Wow, Mom, something weird just happened," Kate says as she gathers our bags. "Jenny just made a new friend." We all laugh; we're being our most generous selves with each other. It's true that I've liked every hospital staff member we've encountered all day, from the woman who took my blood to the radiology tech who gave us the image CD. I'm crowdsourcing prayers, a variety of well wishes, and meaningful handshakes along the way. *People* are making me feel so much better.

For the last appointment of the day, we're led into a small conference room to meet Dr. Darflinger, the doctor who will do tomorrow's embolization. I step out to find the bathroom and stare into the mirror as I wash my hands.

"You're okay," I whisper to the face I've known for thirty-five years. "Keep going. It's all still okay."

But by the time Dr. Darflinger arrives, my head is on the table. I force myself to look up. He's a young guy in green scrubs and a lab coat. We find out he's got a four-month-old daughter who doesn't sleep much at night. It's funny—frightening?—to realize that the doctors who hold your life in their hands might be sleep-deprived from newborns, too.

My mom takes very organized notes and investigates all details.

I let her be the adult and only chime in with childlike questions like *what does it feel like to be put under anesthesia?* and *will I dream?* Dr. Darflinger flips through his file, looking confused.

"I'm sorry, it's just that the notes here say that you're exhibiting a lot of word salad, but I don't find that to be true at all."

"What's word salad?"

"It means that you mix up your language, maybe use different words. But the notes here make it sound like your aphasia is so extreme you can't be understood. I'm going to update your chart."

My eyebrows are on the ceiling. Which ass-clown doctor added these insults to my file? I tell Dr. Darflinger that I'd like to know how I just managed to conduct my vitals in French if I'm so filled with word salad. He laughs. Surprise! I like Darflinger, too.

CHAPTER 8

FOUR DAYS TILL brain surgery. We wake early to get to UCSF ahead of traffic. Today is Embolization Day, and though I'm light on details, the procedure isn't causing anyone else to panic, so I just focus on doing what they tell me.

A nurse hands me a soft gown, points me to a dressing room. When I emerge, she walks us down the muted hall into another room where I hug Chris and my mom in front of the stretcher.

"Good morning, sweetie!" the anesthesiologist says. "Now the first challenge of today is to see if you can climb up on this bed yourself!"

Like a good student, I climb up and follow her instructions about how to position my head. Her eyes are friendly behind the surgical mask, and I wonder who she is when she's not at work.

"I'm going to put a mask over your nose and you'll take a couple big inhales, like a nice big yoga breath. Have you ever done yoga?"

I nod.

"Right, so it's just like that. A couple nice, big breaths. It will smell like a beach ball."

She hovers the mask over my nose and gently holds it steady. I breathe in.

— ⁓ —

Something's pulling on my ears. Gentle pressure. I imagine touching my face to see what it is, but I'm sleepy and warm so I stay how I am.

Now, it's later. Someone's checking on me. I can hear her moving around the room, soft rubber soles on tiled floor. A drawer is opened, then closed. Someone is whispering.

When I open my eyes, the room reassembles. I'm propped up in a bed, wearing an oxygen apparatus. I realize that's what was pulling on my ears. A nurse is leaning over me, Chris is smiling and waving from a chair, and instantly I'm back in my life, back in my body.

I have a brain tumor. The emergency is still happening. The first part is over.

Soft Velcro boots continuously massage my legs to prevent blood clots, and after the nurse checks my vital signs, she removes the oxygen but leaves the tubes hanging from my wrist in case they're needed later. When Dr. Darflinger arrives on rounds, he lingers to explain what just happened.

"We put a tiny coil in an artery in your groin. We fed little beads through blood vessels into your brain so that we could stop the blood flow to the tumor. Because there are so many attachments involved, we wanted to reduce the blood flow to the area as much as we can before surgery."

Chris doesn't seem surprised, which tells me just how much I've been missing while I sit through these appointments. *Beads in my blood vessels?*

"Tomorrow you'll go home and then you'll come back Sunday for another MRI. We want to see how the embolization worked before Dr. McDermott goes in."

Dr. Darflinger logs out of the computer and the original MRI image disappears.

"It's really amazing you found this accidentally," he says. "There's a lot going on in there."

At some point, a doctor will tell me that the tumor was growing for many years, maybe even fifteen, which means that, during my sophomore year at Muhlenberg, a brain tumor sparked. A tiny flame began a long, slow burn. I didn't know. I was busy building a life.

Hot-air balloon rides. College graduation. Shearing sheep. The death of my last grandparent. Teaching English in a small town in rural France, boyfriends, train stations and airports and rental cars, friends' weddings, my wedding, apartment moves and cats and books, so many books. German classes, Spanish classes, yoga classes, writing classes, the beach. Veggie cream cheese on sesame bagels. Betrayals. Making friends, losing friends, finding jobs, leaving jobs, growing babies, birthing babies, sistering, daughtering, wifeing, bossing, mothering. Listening to podcasts while walking over the Brooklyn Bridge.

Fifteen years the fire burned while I filled my gray matter with life experiences, and then one day it had grown so large it started melting down my body's systems. The invisible fire raged. Only I smelled the smoke.

Dr. Darflinger wishes me well and takes his leave. Chris leaves, too. The ICU nurses switch shifts and my new nurse, Lina, props up my pillows. She tracks down a dinner menu.

"Get the ice cream!" she says. "Get two! Why not?"

It's late afternoon on a Friday and for the first time in years, I'm far, far away from what other people are doing at work. Some are on conference calls. Some are finishing presentations. Some are making tough decisions about budgets or layoffs or strategic planning. It occurs to me that none of it actually matters *at all*.

Attentive Lina turns me so that I can watch the sunset while I eat my dinner. The view is so beautiful, the light so warm and easy, that I can tell God is sending me secret, soothing messages.

Hold up. Somehow God snuck in here. Do I now officially believe in God? Foxhole conversion?

Here's a gorgeous sunset in ICU, Jen. Hang in there; I got you.

Maybe it's because I've been spending so much time alone lately, but I've started to sense that something outside myself is interacting with me. An imaginary friend?

This is where my mind is at when Dr. McDermott stops by. I tell him that I'm afraid to go home, knowing that I won't sleep and that the boys will need me. At home, my bedroom is dark and there is no Lina.

"You would need a really good medical reason to stay two more nights," he says. "And as far as I can see, you're fine to go home tomorrow."

The next day, a hospital aide named Marcus arrives from transport to wheel me to the car. He's a young guy, maybe early twenties. I ask him where he's from. He says nearby.

It must be said: San Francisco is not my jam. It's often cold, always cloudy, and other than visiting tech companies and now hospitals, I rarely find reasons to leave the sunnier side of the bay. Some illogical part of me even believes I wouldn't be in this mess if we'd never moved west.

We wait inside in the lobby because it's drizzling. I tell Marcus I'm originally from New York and he says he's always wanted to go. I tell him he should, that there are lots of hospitals in New York.

He says he also wants to go to Jamaica, mostly for the weed.

Be the damn patient, I think to myself. *Not everyone is looking for a career.*

Some phases of a scary medical journey are logistical: commutes, meals, sitting around in waiting rooms. No one includes these scenes in movies because that's not where you find the action. I'm assuming that today's appointment will be similarly boring, a checkup MRI to see how the embolization worked, but I'm wrong about that. Instead of boring, I'm about to stumble into a major life plot twist.

The sun is just starting to rise as we cross the Bay Bridge yet again. This time, my mom stays back with the boys, but Kate is with us. She will wait with Chris while I'm in the tube.

On the third floor, a technician hands me soft green pajamas. When I'm dressed, she walks me into the MRI room and helps me climb up onto the bed. She hands me two yellow foam earplugs and I stuff them in as best I can. Oh, how much has changed since Anthony handed me earplugs two weeks ago! I have graduated to MRI Pro. The technician wraps a cream-colored blanket around my legs. She snaps a plastic mask over my face and pushes me in, a slow descent into the machine's shadows. I'm warm, almost cozy, inside my cocoon.

"Okay, Jennifer, we're going to get started," she says through the speaker. Her voice is a little muffled, scratchy.

"This one will take two minutes." I can barely make out the words, but I don't need the running commentary. Today, there is nothing to do but lie still and wait.

And then, *something unfolds.*

To *unfold.* This is the closest verb I have for what happens, like a version of meditating. I'm awake and calm, not sleeping. I'm not thinking, or pushing or providing direction to my thoughts. Colors emerge and twist and change behind my closed eyes, the way shapes might move inside a lava lamp. For a few moments I'm floating, as if holding a door open for someone. And suddenly I'm watching a scene.

We bought land. Chris is coming into the house; outside, it's misty and I see green, lots of trees and yard.

Another scene. *I'm standing in a construction site, my hand against wooden beams. I'm giving directions. We're building something called Plucky Institute.*

More scenes, more images. *A couple of dogs are running around the land. There are simple housing rooms, rented by clients and companies who come to be on retreat and learn together. Chris is building an experimental unit on the far side of the property. Fruit trees border the yard, visible through the kitchen window while I'm washing dishes.*

The kitchen window is part of the house that we're renovating. Our house shares land with Plucky Institute. We raise our boys here and I walk down the road to work every day.

An interruption.

"Okay, Jennifer, I'm going to come in to give you the contrast now." I'm still in those scenes, but as the technician starts pulling me out, I'm forced back into the bright room.

Plucky Institute? I don't open my eyes; I want back in. The technician injects the substance into my IV port and it spreads icily up my arm.

"Okay, sweetie, only a few more images to go."

Gadolinium-based contrast is running full force through my brain, lighting the path of my blood, but I stay very, very still.

Come back, I think, *come back,* still hungry for whatever that was, but I can't force anything and now the scenes are gone. Despite the obnoxious sounds of the MRI machine, I experience a new quiet, as if someone has just left the room.

Holy shit. Where did all of that come from?

I'm not afraid of dreaming big—I'm a person who not only

dreams of the future, I also construct concrete plans to make it happen. But this, this is different. These are *better* ideas than I've ever had before. As I carefully review these scenes, I receive the most compelling guidance of my life.

You're going to buy land, I hear, but it's not auditory. The message bubbles up from somewhere inside, beyond hearing or feeling, squarely from the realm of conviction.

I know I will live. I know I will teach. I know I will build a physical location for Plucky, that it will be a space and place for humans to connect and grow. I know we will welcome family for extended visits. I know we will be a haven for companies and communities. I see that Plucky is larger than I thought, more than a coaching business, and Plucky Institute is the physical location for its heartbeat.

It feels like I need *days* alone to reflect on what I just experienced, but, of course, the craniotomy train keeps moving. When the technician pulls me out for good, I do normal things like pulling on my jeans and zipping up my sweatshirt, but I am not normal anymore.

Chris is off getting the image CD but Kate is in the waiting room and I decide to confide in her. Kate drinks kombucha. She has a stone Buddha in her backyard. Kate might be the only person in my family who will really believe what just happened.

"I had a vision," I tell her. "I'm going to be fine."

"What vision?"

"I had a vision of our future lives and it involves land and a building, I don't know, something called Plucky Institute. But the big deal is that everything is okay, and I'm going to be okay."

I can tell I'm coming across as weirdly serious, but in this moment, I'm 0 percent self-conscious and 100 percent reassured. When Chris returns, the three of us walk to the parking garage. Well, they walk. I float.

This is a long game, I think. *I still have huge things left to do.*

I have wanted to believe in God my whole life. For thirty-five years, I have been waiting for someone (or something?) to pick up the receiver. People who speak of invisible forces (God, Jesus, spirits, karma, luck, even The Force in Star Wars) also conveniently never know exactly how it works. It seems like unkind or poor planning that God doesn't share a user manual for life, including an FAQ section on how to get in touch. Inconsiderate of an all-powerful being, if you ask me. I have been left to consider two possibilities: either there is a manual and I don't know how to access it. Or there is no God.

These MRI visions allude to a manual. At the very least, I'm aware of something greater than my cognitive functions. My proof is not only the fact that new ideas arrived, fully formed, in my mind. My proof is the indescribable feeling that it was larger than myself, I know it was not me. I am brave and I am smart, but I'm not as hugely, creatively ambitious as the shit that just came out of my tumor-laden brain.

Something bigger is out there, I think. *Okay, Bigness, okay. I finally hear you. What else do you want to say?*

CHAPTER 9

COMMOTION AT THE front door, then hushed laughter. Steve has arrived from DC.

There's always joy at being reunited, a few quick clever jokes about flights, the awe of seeing nephews who are much bigger than last time. Kate, Steve, and I are grown now and spread out across the country. When we meet up these days it's like picking up the sequel to a favorite novel. What is my brother like today? Has he changed since last time, since college, since he was a little boy? Can I find the original Steve in there?

Through the bedroom door, I hear murmurs in the kitchen, a sign that they're talking about me. Everything is so awkward now. How do you make small talk when you might die? Or when you think you won't die because hey, maybe God is real?

I could imagine us laughing about it. *This is crazy weird!* But a brain tumor and brain surgery is *serious* weird, and I'm not even sure what's okay to laugh at anymore. Plus I haven't seen Steve in months; he just got off a plane and maybe underneath it all, I really can't bear to see my little brother cry. I don't want to make any of my family members more sad or worried than they already are, so I stay quiet in the bedroom and pretend to sleep.

After a while, there's a gentle knock at the door and Chris pokes his head in.

"Steve's here."

I blink slowly, as if I'm waking up.

"Okay."

He pushes the door open and they all bound in, my mom, Kate, Steve, Chris, and the boys. They are wearing bright purple T-shirts that say "We Are Plucky!" My mom approaches my side of the bed and shows me pictures of my dad, Steve's wife, and Kate's husband, all wearing purple shirts, too. Steve had them designed and printed.

"We're going to wear these tomorrow!" Mom says.

I'm touched and overwhelmed—but also annoyed. A team of cheerleaders just interrupted my space, and I feel like I have to smile and look grateful even though I don't want to look anything, I want to be depressed and/or ponder mystical visions. Of course, I smile and try to look grateful. Grumpy grateful.

I tell everyone that I want to stay in bed while they prepare for the meal train to arrive. A good friend brings an entire Israeli meal—appetizers and main courses and drinks and desserts. She doesn't stay long, but I make an appearance to receive a hug and a reminder that my body is strong and that I can do anything. Yeah, yeah, yeah. I've heard it all before.

Someone adds the extra leaf to our kitchen table so now it's Thanksgiving, except really, really not. Noah sits to my right and we pass large family-style platters around. Everyone was so lively earlier, chatting easily, but now that I'm here, everything's tense and uncomfortable. Most of the sounds are of people chewing and serving spoons scraping plates. The Last Supper, indeed.

Finally, I excuse myself back to the bedroom where no one can see me. Like the night before a race, I'm wishing we could just speed through to the starting line. I find the same bag I took to the hospital when Aaron was born only nine months ago and start packing: pajamas, underwear, a button-down shirt for the ride home. (Who knows what state my head will be in?) Alone and brash, I grab a pair of scissors from my desk, grip a chunk of my shoulder-length hair, and chop. Voilà, the souvenir from my first thirty-five years. Into a ziplock bag you go.

Should I bring lucky objects? I don't have crosses or clovers or pictures of angels. My eyes scan the room and land on a greeting card I hung up months ago for inspiration.

Do the thing you think you cannot do.

"Pretty good, Eleanor Roosevelt," I say to no one. "I bet you never knew you were talking to brain tumor patients."

The card comes off the wall, goes into my bag. So too does a photo of the four of us from last year's Christmas card and some Scotch tape. Now I'm almost ready.

How do you prepare to leave your children, possibly for the last time? I suppress my nervous energy long enough to sit at my desk. This task is worth my intention.

I don't know what will happen tomorrow, but it seems selfish to simply *assume* the best, so I dig out some envelopes from an old stationery set. When traveling for Plucky, I always leave a daily envelope with a note and stickers for the kids. Aaron is too young to get anything out of it, but it helps Noah track the days until I'm home again. I write notes for seven envelopes, Monday through Sunday. I try to keep things light.

"Did you see any bugs on the playground at school today? Remember and tell Nana or Daddy about them tonight!"

"Can you make a long train with 6 cars? What about 9? Could you drive it all the way back to your bedroom?"

I hold the eighth, yellow envelope in my hands for a long time. I don't write a date on the outside. Instead, I write *To Noah and Aaron* and draw a rainbow. This is the "what if" envelope. My hand hovers over the card. What would Harry Potter's mom have written if she'd known what was going to happen and had time to prepare? *I love looking at the stars,* I write. *Let's always look at them together.*

I draw stars all over the card. If I die, they can have the night sky and, with this note, they will find me there. I tuck this one behind Sunday's envelope and hand the stack to my mom.

"These are for the next seven days," I say. "And, there's one in the back if takes longer."

I leave it at that.

CHAPTER 10

MONDAY, APRIL 25, 2016. Seventeen days since diagnosis. Surgery is scheduled for 12:50pm, and when we arrive at UCSF, we're told to settle into the waiting room on the first floor. The automatic doors keep opening, letting in the chilly San Francisco air, and I'm freezing, curled up on a chair between Chris and my mom. Steve sits nearby. I haven't been allowed to eat or drink since midnight, and the longer we wait, the more irritated I'm getting. In my head, I beg the neurosurgeons to call me up to the OR.

Friends and family, even strangers are thinking of me. Chris shows me a text from his coworker, whose mother lit a candle for me at church in Ireland. Very kind. Another text, this time from my client, whose wife gave birth that very morning. I hold Chris's phone to stare at a fresh, pink baby. I breathe his hopeful newborn energy into my own heart, wondering where little Pete came from, where he was just before he arrived here on earth. *Am I going there today?*

For hours, we wait. Finally around one in the afternoon, Chris says he's going to check with the desk to see what's going on.

"They say that the OR is still in use and they're going to start your surgery a little late."

"Well, can I have a fucking sip of water?"

He checks with the desk; no.

Across from us, a transport aide and an old man in a wheelchair are awaiting discharge papers. It's Marcus!

"HEY, I know you!"

Marcus looks confused. He is a greater character in my story than I in his.

"Remember, we talked about New York? And Jamaica?"

"Oh yeah!"

"Well, it would be *great* to get some New York pizza up in here!" I say. "I can't have food, no drinks, and now my brain surgery is running late."

Marcus's patient looks sympathetic and I reach over to high-five him.

"We should order some rebel patient takeout, me and you!"

Across the room, a woman observes our interactions.

"I don't blame you for being hungry," she says quietly.

Marcus wheels his patient through the exit and I'm back to waiting. Eventually, a woman in a white lab coat calls my name.

"YES!" I declare loudly. "Let's go."

In this moment, all I feel is momentum to get into surgery, which is the biggest blessing of this drug-induced insomnia, because I have no energy for sentimentality. My boys are safe at home, my business is closed, my family is here, and I've been called upstairs to the operating room, where they are going to change my life.

I step firmly into the elevator as the woman leading us presses the button. The door closes.

———

Someone has written *Dary* in green next to *OR room 21* on the whiteboard. Another someone hands me papers to sign, permission slips for the surgery. Shit is getting real.

My prep area, enclosed by a curtain, is small and temporary. They hand me a purple gown and yellow socks to wear. (In ICU, I will look at my feet from my good eye and think about the fact that these socks are the only things that stayed with me from Before to After.) This department has a busy vibe, nurses filling out paperwork and asking questions, disappearing and reappearing around curtains. Soon, the man of the hour arrives.

Dr. McDermott will later ask if I remember what I said to him in OR prep. I do not.

"You said, 'All right, McDerm, let's get this fucking thing out of my head!'" Yup. Sounds exactly like me.

He's holding a clipboard and signing paperwork when I ask him to please shave my whole head while I'm in the OR. He laughs, maybe quizzically, as if full haircuts aren't standard procedure. Normally he would only shave the front few inches of hair.

"Dude, who wants a mullet at this point? I told my kid I wanted to match his little boy hair. Also, I'm not planning to ever do this again, so it's basically a once-in-a-lifetime shaved-head opportunity."

Dr. McDermott gives in, but now he's back to business. He tells Chris he'll call him during the surgery to give updates, says he'll see me in the OR, and leaves.

Here is where I'll make a comment about my surgeon's presence. Dr. McDermott not only conveyed that he had seen it all before and was 100 percent confident about chopping open one's skull; he had a very easy air about him. He never bragged, but he also wasn't a saint. He smiled at my jokes and answered questions matter-of-factly. I was there for brain surgery, yes, but given the kind of work I normally do, I also felt like a secret spy at the hospital, auditing the experience of everyone who worked there. I could see that Dr. McDermott believed in what he and his team could do. As his patient, this gave me an enormous amount of confidence—to the point that I felt relatively calm.

A young anesthesiologist comes in to get several IVs going in my left arm and I look away as she gets to work. My mom watches, chatting about the way the doctors insert needles. I don't understand much of their clinical conversation, but I get the impression based on my mom's reactions that one of the IV lines was the Big One. It sounds like the doctor has just added a loading dock for giant trucks into my left forearm. This idea awakens the first moment of panic, but I keep it to myself. I don't want to push my family's anxiety to frantic levels.

Chris will later tell me that my mom ordered a *shrimp* dish in the hospital cafeteria while I was in surgery and kept commenting on how delicious the *chicken* was. Their stress was real.

Another anesthesiologist arrives and it's time to say goodbye. I'm not entertaining anything but "See you later!" energy. Mom and Chris head downstairs to meet Steve in the waiting room, and now it's time to for me to go, too. The anesthesiologists pop the brakes, pushing my stretcher through the white hallways. Now I'm nervous. I'm also still okay. They hit a button, two doors open simultaneously; they wheel me through and we are surrounded by a small team of nurses and doctors preparing the OR. Everyone is upbeat, jovial, kind. One introduces herself, then a man across the room yells, "Hey! I'm Chef!"

"Hi, super team, I'm Jen! Thanks for taking care of me today!" I have to climb onto another bed and leave my stretcher behind. My stomach spins.

During surgery, they will put a tube in my lungs so I can breathe. Just as with the embolization, the anesthesiologist reminds me that they are giving me 100 percent oxygen for a few minutes and that it's going to smell like a beach ball. Several doctors stand over me and discuss the medication they're going to give, names and amounts that I don't understand.

I'm someone's project, I realize as they put the oxygen mask over my nose and mouth. *I'm what these people are working on today.* This idea is so strange that I'm instantly shy about being the focus of the room and I'm glad I won't be awake during surgery.

Chef is preparing tools. It sounds like Home Depot over there, clinks and bangs of saws, other tools I have no wish to imagine. Now the fear shows up big-time and I'm trying to focus on the oxygen mask and not notice the nurses and doctors crowding into the room. *What the ever-loving fuck is about to happen to me?* Panic rising, I want to say something but the oxygen mask is already working and I don't want to disrupt the project and I really, really want this surgery to be done so I can move on with my beautiful, visioned life so I do the only thing that comes to mind: I sing quietly in my head.

This little light of mine, I'm going to let it shine.
This little light of mine, I'm going to let it shine.
This little light of mine, I'm going to let it shine.
Let it shine, shine, shine, let it . . .

And before I finish the verse, I'm gone.

PART II

CHAPTER 11

IT IS DARK. I am in a bed.

"Honey, we're here," someone whispers. Sounds familiar. I open my eyes.

All around me, stagehands have changed the scenery. The Operating Room props have been put away; now we are in quiet ICU where little lights glow and soft machines are humming.

Maybe it's nighttime?

The three Loved Ones are in this scene, figures standing along the bed, holding jackets and tote bags.

Husband whispers, "You're out of surgery!"

I've forgotten my line. What am I supposed to say next?

"Everything went so well, it couldn't have gone better!" Husband is talking much too fast but sounds convincing. "McDermott says Simpson Grade 1."

Simpson Grade 1. I remember a piece of this story. Brain tumor? It's out?

"Oh!" I say. "Okay."

Mother steps forward, puts her hand on my leg. "Sweetie, you did so well! He got the whole thing out."

Maybe they will know I'm okay if I say something.

"Okay."

Male Nurse appears from stage left. He is checking something, maybe related to my arm. He trades dialogue with The Loved Ones. Brother hangs back.

"We have to leave because it's late," Husband says. "But we'll be back in the morning. I love you, you're amazing."

"Thanks."

He squeezes my hand, then steps toward the door.

Mother rubs my leg again. "Get some rest, you're going to feel better in no time!"

Brother steps toward the bed and pats my hand. "Love you," he whispers.

The Loved Ones are gone. Male Nurse is gone. I close my eyes.

———

Awake again. Same scenery. ICU is quiet, very dark. My head is bandaged and I am propped up on many pillows. Male Nurse comes in.

"Hello, Jennifer," he says. "I'm Ron. I'm going to be your nurse tonight."

Nurse Ron moves quietly around the room, checking, connecting, disconnecting attachments to my body.

"To call me, press this button." He puts the remote in my hand. "I'm right outside."

His is a comforting message.

———

I am waking up. I am quiet and dull but I am still me. A relief.

The next time Nurse Ron comes into the room, I call him over.

"I need to tell you something." My voice is scratchy.

"Yes, of course. What is it?" Nurse Ron has an accent.

"I had a vision in the MRI machine. It came from something very big, maybe something like God. I saw my future."

"Oh my! What was your future?" Nurse Ron leans in.

It feels important to say these things out loud.

"I can't remember all the details right now, but I'm going to buy land and build a center for learning. I'm going to get people together."

"Wow! I believe you will, Jennifer!"

Nurse Ron, my champion! I want to hear him say he believes in the vision again and again.

"Keep dreaming of that; that's a beautiful future," he says. He hands me a few pills to swallow with some water. "Now try to rest."

He shows me the remote again and returns to his spot behind the glass.

I am simple in ICU. *I know myself.* In my bed, in the dark, with the machine lights blinking, I am padded away from the rest of the world, as if I am in space, as if everyone else is far, far away breathing different air.

In this seemingly empty room, I feel so loved.

In this dark room, I am love.

I allow Nurse Ron to keep my body safe but I don't want anyone else to come. I want to stay here with the greater presences that I can't see or name but who are fully holding and watching over me. The room is thick with protection.

I am not alone.

⌒

The MRI visions are close. Someone is here, holding and attending to their message. Who?

It's not Jesus or God or someone so intimidating. Maybe a spiritual social worker was assigned to my case. Who's in charge of my file?

A sort of angel representative, I think. She broke the fourth wall during the MRI by showing me the slide deck of my future. I wonder if she was supposed to do that or if she went rogue. I hope she's a rebel. I hope she breaks more rules for me.

I'm listening, I think, staring into the dark corner of the room. *When you can share more, I'm ready.*

I imagine her smiling to her invisible self and crossing off a task on her professional angel clipboard.

Initial connection: CHECK.

⌒

Before sunrise, a young, dark-haired doctor comes in, pulling on purple gloves as he moves. Reluctantly, I give up the quiet of the room.

"Hi there, Ms. Dary, I'm Dr. Michael Safaee." He pulls out a flashlight, which he uses to look in my right eye. Then he pulls open my left eye, which is swollen shut. I guess I've been a cyclops since surgery; I hadn't noticed.

"Is there blurriness?" he asks. I don't know.

"Is there pain?" Again, I am at a loss.

I can tell he is trying to rule out symptoms of something, but I can't guess what.

"The swelling is going to get worse before it gets better," he says, writing on a chart.

Well if that isn't inspirational! I think. Who is this efficient, blunt doctor? My curiosity brings me back to conversational.

"Hey, are you from around here?"

"Los Angeles."

Figures.

———

The next time he comes in the room, Dr. Safaee snaps on his gloves and advances toward the bed. I am ready.

"Well, well, well . . . if it isn't Dr. Mike from LA." Clearing my throat, I make the sentence crawl, as if we're old friends meeting at a bar. This time he pauses and almost smiles.

"How are you, Jennifer?" He takes out his flashlight to look at my swollen mess, but through my good eye I can tell I have softened him.

"What's going on with this eye?" I ask. "What are you checking for?"

"Blurriness. It's a sign that the eye could have been damaged during surgery, but your vision will also be blurry while it heals, so it's hard to tell."

We talk a little more and then he says he has to go check someone else's eyeball-brain connection.

"Peace out, Dr. Mike from LA," I call softly as he's leaving. He waves.

———

Now, the sun is up. Nurse Ron is gone and the room feels less protected. The daytime ICU nurses say I can order food, so I look over the menu with one eye. Waffles, pancakes, yogurt, all sorts of omelets. My approved options are more limited though and, oddly, the left side my mouth doesn't open anymore, so I order scrambled eggs. As soon as I've ordered, the daytime nurses say I need to go down for an MRI. No one is clear about timing here—will eggs or transport get here first? Two hours later, transport still hasn't arrived, but I also haven't been cleared to eat yet. My cold eggs lie on the tray. The sunlight is harsh in the room, intruding. Can't someone close the FUCKING drapes?

People are kinder to nice patients, I know, so I'm trying to play along, but I haven't eaten in days and my mouth is broken. I miss Nurse Ron; the daytime nurses are busy, they don't have time to listen, and I don't even *want* to tell them about my life-changing spiritual experiences. Hmph.

"Why is my mouth so tight?" I ask Daytime Nurse when she comes into the room.

"The surgeons had to detach your left temporalis muscle and remove some eye bone and cheekbone during surgery," she says, moving objects around the room. "They reattached it and put it back, but it will take some time before you can use it easily again."

No one told me they were detaching muscles and taking out eye bone and cheekbone. Did they put it all back?!

"Can I at least eat?"

The nurse pushes the tray over to my bed and I try to gently push minuscule egg blobs through the right corner of my mouth, slow work. Of course, transport arrives at that very moment. Two guys disconnect me from machines before moving my bed away from the eggs and toward the elevator. I'm pissed that they haven't apologized for their lateness or that they'd interrupted my breakfast. I wonder what they would be talking about in the elevator if I wasn't there. I feel invisible, a social inconvenience.

When we get to the imaging room the technician helps me move carefully off of my bed. This is my first time upright since surgery. My skull feels like a bunch of jigsaw pieces, loose, untrustworthy. Opening my jaw to speak makes me feel like it might not close back up, as if the bones are too fragile and they don't work together anymore. Now I'm climbing onto a new stretcher, now I'm settling into the head rest, now I'm plugging my ears with earplugs stained by blood oozing from the incision. My IV has extra-long tubing so the metallic pole can stay outside the door and won't mess with the machine.

"Okay, Jennifer, we're going to get started," the technician says through the speaker.

Bumps and bangs and screeches from the machine add to the hellish atmosphere. I can tell there will be no life-changing visions this time around. I invite patience to flood my mind.

Yo, angel rep, call Customer Service, I think. *I am low.*

———

After the MRI, the tech says that transport is ready to take me back to ICU. The door opens and in strolls Marcus.

"I can't believe it!" I'm broken-mouth gaping at him. In the movie version, Marcus would gasp and cry a few nostalgic tears, but real-life Marcus doesn't recognize me. To be fair, my head has been shaved. My left eye is shut and my face is swollen from steroids and all the surgeons realigning my face bones.

"Remember me? We talked about New York in the waiting room . . . yesterday."

Yesterday. How could so much have changed in 24 hours?

"Oh yeah . . ." He trails off and nods in my direction. His partner hits the elevator button, indifferent to our reunion. By the time we get back to my room in ICU, Marcus's voice has warmed up from "totally bored" to "more or less human." He tells me to feel better soon.

The cold eggs are gone, but I do feel a little more alert. In a hospital as large at UCSF, I take these Marcus coincidences as my angel rep signaling.

Keep going, I imagine her saying. *We haven't left you. Magic is still here.*

———

I'm to be transferred out of ICU, but first Chris and Kate come to visit. Daytime Nurse suggests getting me up for a walk. As they help me out of bed, I see that the TV in my room has been on all night. Unable to lift even my good eye, I hadn't realized I'd turned it on.

The nurse steers me toward a large window overlooking the Bay Bridge and Golden Gate Park. Chris and Kate keep saying, "Wow! How pretty is this view, this hospital is like a hotel!" Here is our first differentiator: I can't see views because I can't focus on anything but my own next step. My body is slow and limited, so I leave them at the window and, with the nurse's help, shuffle back to bed.

Later I will find out what really happened in surgery. Later I will understand, even research, the process of detaching someone's temporalis muscle, a circular muscle that goes from the back of your eyes to the area above your ear. You need it for chewing.

What did it look like when they lifted my chewing muscle and glimpsed my skull? And then when they sawed holes in it, took out pieces of my bones, placed them carefully on a tray for a while—a few minutes or was it hours?—while they kept digging toward the tumor?

Once, a dentist asked Chris where he grew up. The dentist could tell something about his teeth based on the water in Wisconsin. The places we live and the things we've experienced can mark us in ways that are only visible to some.

It's so wild that my inside parts, the muscles and bones that truly keep me alive, are least known to me. I wonder what story my skull tells about where I grew up. In quiet moments, I daydream about Dr. McDermott carving his initials into my skull. *McDermott wuz here. UCSF Neuro 4eva.* In this way, Dr. McDermott will remain one of the most intimate people in my life. After recovery, I will not share a word with him in person for years, but he is in my closest mental circle. McDermott has seen parts of me that no one—not even I—will ever see.

CHAPTER 12

"DO YOU WANT me to wipe some of these eye boogers?" Nurse Elisha has taken charge of me, now that I've been transferred to the Neuro unit. Nurses talk differently to me on the eighth floor.

"Yeah," I say. "Please."

"Eye boogers" is the most accurate phrase I've heard lately, and Elisha is my new favorite person because suddenly I can't find language for *anything*. All I sense is discomfort, exhaustion, heavy energy weighing me down, but I don't know how to express this in words. Elisha translates me to myself.

For a while, I have a catheter but once they remove it, I need to call for help to get to the bathroom. "DO NOT THINK ABOUT GETTING OUT OF BED ALONE," nurses order again and again. McDermott—I am told—is infamous for keeping his neuro patients well hydrated through bags and bags of fluids, so I'm feeling like a pest with all the bathroom trips.

Here is how you plan peeing in the hospital: Call the nurses' station to ask for help. Wait for a nurse to come. Take the blankets off. Wait for the nurse to detach your legs from the blow-up booties preventing blood clots. Swing your legs over the side of the bed, try to stand up. Wait for the nurse to move the IV stand. Grab the IV stand and roll it slowly alongside you as the nurse walks behind offering—when needed—a supportive hand on your back. Wait for the nurse to put the pee bucket in the toilet so she can measure output. Shakily sit on the toilet. Pee. Ask the nurse to return. Wait. Let her help you up. Wash your hands. Slump across the room. Sit. Get into bed and reconnect everything in reverse order. The process is tiring, but I'm proud of peeing so many cc's.

Listen, the achievement bar on the eighth floor is low.

⁓

Ema, my new roommate, is twenty years old and she's in the hospital because of complications with a pituitary tumor. This means that she is barely peeing, not allowed to drink water, and required to take salt tablets. It sounds like *hell*. I learn all of this through the curtain that divides our room. She is really mad at her mom, who keeps talking, and, understandably, Ema has a really bad headache.

During one of her checks, Elisha helps me tape the small wallet-size family picture on the railing of my bed. I wasn't allowed to hang anything on the walls in ICU, but the eighth floor is different, kind of like a dorm room. I consider calling Ema over to say hi and show her the picture of the kids, if only to give her a break from her own family, but I don't have the energy to speak louder than a whisper. I close my eyes and listen to their family dynamics, as if they are a television show playing in the background. I hold Radish, my stuffed pink rabbit, close. Sometimes I doze off for a few minutes or force my only working eyelid open so I can see my Eleanor Roosevelt card, which Elisha pinned to the corkboard near my bed.

Do the thing you think you cannot do, says Eleanor.

I am, I think, many times an hour. *I'm here, existing.*

I live in a bubble. Time moves slowly.

With long flowing blond hair, she looks like a lady from a Mucha painting. We first hear Jennifer Viner's name in McDermott's office at our initial visit, but I don't meet her until she sweeps into room 831, a nurse practitioner with purpose in her step. She approaches the bed, confidently dabs at the blood on my surgical wound, as if she is certain it won't hurt. And it doesn't.

"How's it going, Smurfette?" She adjusts my head bandages.

"Okay." It's the best answer I've got. With nothing to compare this experience to, I can't see forward or reflect back. I seem to be alive.

There are some people who make you feel better just by being in the same room. Jennifer Viner is one of those people. I don't know if it's her energy or the strength of her experience, but being with her feels electric. As she checks my chart, looks intently at my swollen eye, she is totally concentrated. I can tell she doesn't want to be anywhere else. It is so rare to feel like you're receiving 100 percent of someone's attention, and I quietly decide to make people feel like this as often as I can when I'm out of this mess.

I'm dying to ask Jennifer Viner coaching questions about her love of neurology and how many patients she's seen so far today and what she does to relax after such a stressful job. This hospital is suddenly as stimulating to me as a huge city, filled with McDermotts and Jennifer Viners and Dr. Mikes from LA and beyond, each staff member and patient on their own journey. But tracking people's stories is not my work today, so I hold Radish tight to my chest and let Jennifer take care of me.

After she leaves the room, I wonder why she called me Smurfette. I can feel my swollen eye; I know I have no hair. But what do I look like?

Getting to a mirror is out of the question, so I open my phone's camera app and turn the view around, as if to take a selfie.

First impression: a figure, in shadows, white gauze covering its head.

Comprehension readjusted: a chubby, ugly head, vaguely familiar nose and lips, one eye peering back at the lens. This head is foreign, so strange that I almost expect it to start talking back at me, independently. *Am I inside of that?*

I'm not sad about my swollen face or bright purple eye or the loss of my hair—not yet, anyway. Instead, I'm weirdly fascinated.

I'm living this and *I'm observing it.*

I'm the main character and *the story's narrator.*

I'm more than what is seen and *more than what I think.*

This is what it means to be alive.

⁓

The Loved Ones have come to visit me on the eighth floor. They enter the room, whispering. I keep my eyes closed, more tired than I've ever been, but also guilty to have put them through terrible Bay Bridge traffic just to watch me sleep. I've not yet figured out how to be grateful and antisocial. I wish the nurses would put me into a forced-sleep state so I could rest and not host. But, real talk, there is no way to track how far out of the proverbial woods I am yet, so I live constantly on edge. What else might the doctors find? I'm aware of the importance of everything, every word and gesture, every moment between us.

Will you tell this story at my funeral? Will you tell my sons about this moment, one day, long from now when they ask their family for any memories of their mom before she was a vegetable, the version of a woman who they barely remember? Do I have it in me to make one more memory for you to pass on to my boys?

After a few minutes of watching me rest, my mom and Chris go to get drinks and Steve holds my hand. I can't remember the last time that happened. My little brother. I open my eyes. For him.

Let me tell you what holding your younger brother's hand in the hospital feels like. You feel really old, like you've warp-sped into the future when you're in a nursing home and someone's visiting you, delicately. You're the older one who has always been the backbone, but now you're feeble and you use whatever energy you can to make a joke or deflect from the dramatic situation you all find yourselves in. You have your first honest post-op laugh with him when he says my greeting should be "You think I look bad? You should see the other guy!"

Every time your mom enters the room, she says, "Your eye is looking so much better! You'll see, you're going to be feeling more like yourself in no time!"

Your husband seems nervous and worried and tired; still, you know he's got everything under control because he is the most dependable person you know.

Your sister stops by between UCSF classes, and you offer to share your saltines with her because she's only a few weeks pregnant with the person who'll be your first niece, and she's nauseous. She sits on the windowsill and you talk about your wounds, make jokes about the Kardashians, grateful for the calm energy she brings. The next nurse that arrives to help you to the bathroom meets your sister and announces, "You two look so much alike!"

You both laugh. Since your head is shaved and you look like someone beat your face with a frying pan, this is the best compliment you've ever received.

⁓

Ema leaves early in the evening. She has requested a private room and is wheeled out, parents following closely behind. I try not to take offense—maybe my constant peeing has made her jealous?—and I rest as the staff cleans her side of the room. When Elisha comes in to give me my night meds, she tells me to enjoy the quiet for a while. A few soft lights from the nearby machines keep me company. I'm looking forward to a long, deep sleep as the solo occupant of room 831.

But sleep doesn't come. Instead, I spin.

I'm scheduled to go home the next day, but I want to stay here. Barely out of surgery, it's unclear what my body can and can't handle outside this hospital. I haven't slept more than an hour consecutively in days, and I don't know how to define this new reality, let alone manage it. But what I think about most are the boys.

How will Noah react to the way I look? Will he be scared of his mom? For a while I weigh the pros and cons of wearing a hat or a scarf. Or sunglasses? I wonder if we should FaceTime before he sees me in person? Maybe it would drastically lower his expectations and give him time to process this with my mom and Chris before I get home. I feel pressure to get this arrival right, exerting a little control amidst the chaos.

And Aaron. I won't be allowed to carry anything heavier than five pounds for a couple weeks, which means I can't hold my son. Aaron is our brute, a very determined, very physical guy, known for being rough and active. How am I going to have any kind of relationship with him, knowing that he might clock me in the broken head at any moment? Will he want to nurse? Will he cry when he sees my face? I couldn't bear it if he did.

It is one thing to be tended to in a hospital where people are paid to care for you. It is quite another to return to a home where two young kids dictate the schedule and tempo of the small space. I worry about Chris feeling torn between his responsibilities to each of us, and I worry about what we'll do when Steve goes back to DC.

Here on the eighth floor, wearing a hospital gown, no one expects anything of me, but how long can I hold off others' expectations at home? And, let's be honest: I'm not even sure if I can trust my own abilities to let guilt and expectations stay on the sidelines. What if I'm trying to pack lunches by Monday? I haven't had caffeine in days—still I'm amped up and wide awake. Elisha arrives with the next dose of painkillers, a welcome interruption.

"Hey there," she calls softly. "Did you get any sleep?"

"Not yet. I'm feeling pretty awake. Kind of nervous."

"Got it," she says. "I think there's a meditation channel on this TV thing. Want to try it?"

She flips through the channels but can't find it so she tucks me in, makes sure Radish is in my arms, and leaves me to rest again. After a few minutes I try the white noise app we use when we stay in hotels, but even on the lowest volume, the sounds of soft rain are brutal on my brain, so I turn it off and try to sit with the silence of the room, breathing slowly in and out, in and out. *There's no rush,* I think. *There's nothing to wake up for; sleep as long as you can.*

I'm just starting to feel sleepy when I hear a commotion in the hall. Someone new is coming.

———

"Ten out of ten!" someone is screaming. "TEN OUT OF TEN! No relief. None! There's NO relief!"

The patient is wheeled into Ema's old spot shortly after midnight, followed by at least four nurses. I can't see anything through the curtain, only the staff as they come in and out of the room. They are hooking up machines as the woman wails and demands pain meds over and over and over again.

The story that I catch is that she's been waiting in the ER since noon. Her family kicked her out because she hasn't been able to manage the pain on her own at home, and they are tired of hearing about it. UCSF makes patients say their name and birth date fifty times a day, so I quickly learn that her name is Nadia and that she is one year younger than me.

"The pain never stops!" Nadia cries. The nurse administers pain meds and comes back a few minutes later to see if they're helping.

"No!" she cries, "it's just as bad as before, it's worse than before! I need more pain medication; if I can't get it here I'll have to leave and go to another hospital!"

Good idea! I think.

"Please! Help me!" Nadia screams. "Ten out of ten, ten out of ten!" I'm fully awake listening to this, completely convinced that she doesn't have ten-out-of-ten pain.

Am I going to have to coach this girl through the curtain? I wonder. I consider telling her about the Eleanor Roosevelt quote on my bulletin board, but remind myself that I'm on medical leave from Plucky and, oh, I've just had brain surgery myself so maybe best to let those on duty handle things?

Around 3am, the doctor on call comes in to speak with her. They discuss dosages of some medicine; whatever she's suggesting must be extreme because the doctor tells her they have to be careful, what she's asking for is what killed Michael Jackson.

Good lord, I think. *Who is this person? And how can these nurses and doctors be staying so calm in the face of what must be a drug addiction?*

The doctor writes the order for the drugs and Nadia continues moaning for a while. I write her off, hoping she'll be transferred to the psychiatric ward in short order. Eventually, I fall asleep, though I continue to be woken up by nurses when they come in to check on one of us every half hour.

When Chris gets to UCSF the next day, he overhears the name of her condition: Acute Intermittent Porphyria (AIP). We look it up online and are horrified to read that this very rare condition *does* cause the dramatic pain levels that Nadia was describing. She wasn't being dramatic; she was ten out of ten! Again I'm reminded that you just never know anybody else's truth. It takes a lot to be grateful for brain surgery. Home is now sounding more appealing.

～

I'm thinking about Anthony, my original MRI tech from April 8. The machine wasn't broken—this must have been his excuse to get me across the hall without arising suspicion. Anthony saw the tumor first.

And now I'm remembering the female technician who asked if I'd been having headaches and the other people who were in the room when they pulled me out of the tube. They all knew, too.

I remember how I joked with Anthony on my way to the locker to retrieve my shoes.

"That wasn't so bad!" I'd said.

I replay this scene over and over in my head, each time hearing my words with their tragic underlay, perhaps the way Anthony heard them.

Before 8am on April 8, 2016, Anthony had seen a large tumor inside a young mother's brain. With this knowledge, he kindly moved her to a different machine and coached her through the rest of the images. I assume he continued on all day, conducting MRIs for some patients who found problems and for others whose health was cleared. Maybe after work he cut someone off in traffic or was short with a barista or yelled at a customer service representative who refused his refund.

I'm swooping across the city, the state, the world, watching these moments take place on April 8. *But you don't understand,* I want to tell each person who may have experienced conflict with Anthony. *He had a deeply sad day.* I see how every interaction affects every other interaction and like a map, I can walk the path to each outcome and forgive both sides. From this bed on the eighth floor, I can see that everything has impact. Every single event has consequence.

CHAPTER 13

IN A FEW hours Chris and Mom will arrive to bring me home, but first they are compiling a shopping list. Shower stool. Pill box. Wedge pillow. Lap tray.

The physical therapists are here to take me on a walk. We circle the floor twice and then we move into a stairwell so I can practice stepping up and down a few stairs. After three times, I'm too wiped to continue, so the PTs walk me back to my bed as we talk about what it will be like at home.

"It's really important to scan the area ahead of you," one PT says. "Since one of your eyes is out of commission for a while, you'll need to turn your head back and forth so you can use your right eye. You don't want to fall!"

I imagine the home I'm heading back to, an ever-changing obstacle course. Trains, toys, cats, shoes, backpacks, a crawling baby. In my UCSF eighth-floor bubble, I'm protected. Home sounds like the neuro version of *Ninja Warrior*.

Back in room 831, Jennifer Viner is here to say good morning.

"What's all this?" she asks, pointing to a rash on my face and chest.

Nurses have been mentioning it each time they take me to pee. "Oh, sweetie, you're getting a rash on your back!" they say as they support me from behind.

I don't care. I have bigger issues than some rash, notably the fact that *I must be accompanied to pee,* but by the look on Jennifer's face, I'm guessing the rash is finally a big deal. She requests a dermatology consult and tells me I can't be discharged until I see them. They arrive a few hours later, two women in white lab coats.

The dermatologists circle me and ask if they can look at and touch various areas of my body. Today, I'm their specimen. They are fascinated and ask to take pictures. Listening to them is like being in a foreign country, dermatological vocabulary flying, and I'm grateful that they're talking to each other and not to me. I barely have the energy to speak more than two syllables.

At the end of the dermatologists' sleuthing, Dr. McDermott and Jennifer Viner arrive and the group digests my case for a few minutes. It's like observing National Geographic, four mega-experts learning from each other in the UCSF wild. Jennifer Viner reads the list of my allergies aloud, specifically a family of antibiotics. McDermott asks high-level questions and listens intently as the dermatologists explain the connections. It turns out the antibiotic I received during surgery was in the same family and I was pumped full of it. Now I'm having one massive allergic reaction.

All of this is news to me, of course, because I can't *see* the rash, but then I can't see much of anything at all. When I finally catch the residual hives a week later in my bathroom mirror, the huge spots all over my body are shocking. No wonder those nurses had been commenting; I must have looked like a genuine leopard.

⌒

Nurse Elisha is back on day shift and she keeps checking: Have I pooped yet? You can't leave if you haven't pooped, even if the problematic body part that landed you in the hospital is located very far from your bowels. No, I keep reporting. No, no, not yet, no, sorry. It's midmorning when Elisha brings out the big guns.

"Okay. I have a suppository, Jen—say the word, and we'll get things moving."

Who knows why I'm stubborn about this? Maybe I want my body to wake up and do its own thing, show a sign of normal life without a drug or invasion to prompt it. Chris texts that they're almost ready to leave Berkeley. *See you in a bit!* he says. I imagine the slow-downs they're about to wade through on the bridge while cringing at the traffic we'll face on our way back. I imagine needing to postpone our return by a few hours because I'm being inflexible and not accepting help with the poop problem.

"You know," I grumble up toward the ceiling. "I'm really getting sick of all this required flexibility."

I press the nurse's call button and Elisha pops her head in to see what's up.

"Fine," I tell her. "Make me poop."

⌒

A new nurse, Arma, arrives and decides we can take the port out of my right arm to get me ready for discharge. She removes the port and goes to take the tubes out of my left arm too, but blood is suddenly running down my right arm, dripping on the floor and staining the sheets. Arma gasps and moves quickly to stop the flow. I can see her thinking it through, tracing the lines with her eyes until she realizes that someone in the last shift forgot to put a cap on the port.

The repercussions are immediate. A staff member comes in to change the sheets right away. Someone brings me a new gown. The blood on the floor is cleaned with special fluid by a nurse who dons an official hazmat cleaning suit. As sci-fi as these moments are, I'm not bothered by the sight of my blood. It is so vibrant, so beautiful and deep red. My blood is *alive*.

Later, Dr. McDermott tells me that I didn't lose much blood during brain surgery, a direct result of the embolization.

"How much is not much?"

"About fifty cc."

Fifty cc is slightly more than the medicine cup that comes with Children's Tylenol. Modern medicine is amazing.

⁓

My mom and Chris arrive. We pack up the few items I had with me, unsticking the Eleanor Roosevelt quote and our family picture from the wall. Jennifer Viner and Dr. Mike from LA arrive in room 831 to check me one last time, typing quickly and signing my discharge papers. As they pull off their gloves to leave, I feel massive panic rising in my chest. This can't be the ending!

"Wait!" They pause at the curtain.

What do you say? *How* can you say it? These people have worked tirelessly to keep me and many other patients alive in the four days that I've known them. My gratitude is overwhelming, also inexpressible. I haven't cried a tear since surgery, and despite how awkward it feels considering everyone in the room, I know I'll deeply regret never thanking them.

Later there will be moments when brain surgery seemed much easier than I'd made it out to be. Hindsight, especially when recovery and healing go extremely well, diminishes the darkest moments of our darkest times. But the fact remains that, for over four hours on the afternoon of April 25, 2016, my life was the closest to over that it had ever been. I'm alive today because of science and machines. Very talented doctors and nurses kept my systems functioning while surgeons opened my skull. A tube in my lungs breathed for me. I was the most defenseless that I'd ever been, also more protected than I'd ever been, too.

A tidal wave of emotion constricts my throat as I look up at them, Dr. Mike from LA with his energetic precision and the brilliant Jennifer Viner, with her expert capabilities.

"Thank you," I say. "Thank you for saving my life."

I'm crying, embarrassingly, loud, unstoppable. My mom and Chris turn to comfort me, while Jennifer Viner and Dr. Mike from LA quietly take their exit from the room.

The floodgates won't be fully open for weeks but tears will find ways out, sparked by random moments. This initial burst, however, allows the first release. One eye is swollen shut and my head is still bleeding, but my tear ducts, I realize, are working just fine.

Chris descends to get the car while my mom and I wait for the official paperwork. Arma walks us through the whole thing. We learn that her husband used to work at my mom's company and her daughter used to go to the same daycare as my kids. *What a tiny, tiny world,* I think. *We're all so connected.*

"You were here for the removal of a meningioma of the left sphenoid wing, involving cavernous sinus," she reads from the discharge form. It's strange for the past three days and weeks and years of my life to be summarized so succinctly. Arma walks us through the drugs I need to continue taking and shows my mom how to give me a daily shot in the belly to prevent blood clots. Transport arrives with a wheelchair—sadly, no Marcus this time!—and we are off, heading down the elevator to where Chris is waiting with the car, ready to start our post-op, post-poop lives.

Mom puts me in the front seat and she sits in the back. Everything outside the windows represents a massive amount of information—cars, blinking lights, birds, people in crosswalks, planes overhead—and it's too stimulating, so I close my eyes for the entire drive home. No music, no talking. I breathe in and out, then in and out again. Over and over this is what I focus on, a sort of breath-based conveyor belt, scared to imagine where I will be in an hour, in denial that I'm leaving where I was an hour ago.

———

Jennifer Dary, your discharge medication list is listed below:

Desonide 0.05% cream (for rash)—Apply to the face and neck twice daily.

Dexamethasone 1 mg tablet—Take according to taper calendar. This is a steroid used for brain swelling. Take evenly spaced throughout the day. CALL YOUR DOCTOR for symptoms of: headaches that are not controlled with pain medicine; sedation, confusion, weakness; vision or speech changes.

Triamcinolone 0.1% lotion (for rash)—Apply to the body twice daily.

Cholecalciferol (vitamin D3) 1,000 unit cap—Take 2,000 units by mouth nightly at bedtime.

Docusate sodium 250 mg capsule (for prevention of constipation)—Take 1 capsule (250 mg total) by mouth 2 (two) times daily.

Enoxaparin 40 mg/0.4 mL injection (for preventing blood clots)—Inject 0.4 mLs (40 mg total) into the skin daily. Last dose 5/3/16.

Multivitamin tablet (for wound healing)—Take 1 tablet by

mouth daily. Last dose 5/10/16.

Pantoprazole 40 mg EC tablet (to prevent stomach upset)—Take 1 tablet (40 mg total) by mouth daily while on dexamethasone.

Polyethylene glycol 17 gram packet (for prevention of constipation)—Take 1 packet (17 g total) by mouth daily.

Prenatal multivitamins 28 mg iron-800 mcg tab—Take by mouth nightly at bedtime. Do not take vitamins until 5/10/16, at least 2 weeks from date of surgery.

Senna 8.6 mg tablet (for prevention of constipation)—Take 2 tablets (17.2 mg total) by mouth nightly at bedtime.

Vits A and D-white pet-lanolin ointment (for wound healing)—Apply topically 2 (two) times daily. Last dose 5/10/16.

Take these medications as needed:

Acetaminophen 500 mg tablet (for MILD PAIN)—Take 1 tablet (500 mg total) by mouth every 6 (six) hours as needed.

HYDROcodone-acetaminophen 10-325 mg tablet (for pain)—Take 1-2 tablets by mouth every 4 (four) hours as needed for pain.

Start on 5/10/2016:

LORazepam 1 mg tablet (for anxiety)—Take 1 tablet (1 mg total) by mouth every 8 (eight) hours as needed for anxiety.

CHAPTER 14

WE ARE HOME. Chris helps me up the stairs and into the house. I move slowly, leaning on the back of the blue couch; then against the wooden kitchen table; finally, hands tracing the yellow hallway walls. Now in our room, he helps me into bed. From my good eye, I recognize this setting: framed drawings of Central Park, tall dresser topped with stray jewelry, a stack of novels near my side of the bed. I'm the stranger among familiar objects.

Steve is awaiting the all-clear to bring Noah home from the park, and once I'm settled, Chris texts to say they can come back. I brace for impact, extremely aware that I smell like a hospital.

Noah bounces down the hall, talking about the playground and seeing Mommy. I pool every ounce of energy I have to use a voice louder than a whisper, to seem in good spirits and to make a few jokes. He quickly approaches my side of the bed and pauses when he sees my face.

"Why did they take all your hair?" he asks, his eyes narrowing. I explain that those silly doctors took too much, but that it will grow back fast and soon we'll have matching haircuts. He reaches for the left side of my face, but Chris holds back his little hand.

"Why can't you open that eye?"

Soon we'll have the idea to buy matching pirate eye patches, but for now we explain that I have a boo-boo and it's getting better every day.

"How was school, buddy? Did you play outside today?"

"I don't want to talk about it," he mumbles and heads for the bedroom door.

Kate and Steve immediately come into my room and start chatting, an act that shows Noah that Mom is indeed in there, just looking different.

Everyone says that kids are resilient, but I don't dare to believe it until Noah proves it's true. He's back a few minutes later to check out my new sturdy lap tray, where I'll be eating dinner that night. "Let's play restaurant!" he says and asks to eat his dinner next to me.

I never considered myself a sentimental mom, but in these moments I can't deny the importance of a mother's love. The initial conversation has gone better than I'd hoped—no traumatic screams—and the fact that he's looking past my disfigured exterior to still find me there means *everything*.

But how to translate this experience for a baby?

I'm afraid Aaron will see me, cry, refuse me, and break my heart. Or, the opposite, that he will want more than I can give. I can't bear showing him that I'm home but unable to hold or nurse or soothe him and I'm not allowed to lift more than five pounds for the first few weeks, anyway. I tell Chris to keep him away from me until the next day. Before bed, Chris tells me that Aaron knows Mom is home, that he kept smiling in the direction of our bedroom door. Damn. This fills and breaks and boosts my heart.

My makeshift hospital room rivals the Neuro unit. Chris has installed four night-lights and Mom sets up water and snacks, brings me my evening meds. I keep my phone nearby so I can see the time. I snuggle Radish under our fuzzy beige comforter. I hold out as long as I can before waking Chris to help me pee, because there's no way I'm making it to the bathroom alone. Arma said that my head has to remain elevated so, these first few nights, I must sleep on a wedge pillow. This is so terribly uncomfortable that I can only sleep an hour or two at a time. Even once the wedge is retired, I won't be able to sleep on my left side because my face will still be swollen for many weeks.

I listen to Chris's breathing, to the cats' snoring, to the quiet of the dark. I don't miss having roommates, but it is lonely to be the only one awake all night, so I look my nurses up on LinkedIn. I find Elisha, Arma, Jennifer Viner. Just seeing their faces makes me feel better. For the moment, my angel rep has gone silent. I wish she was on LinkedIn, too.

～

Chris is picking the kids up from daycare. I've been resting most of the afternoon, reserving all my energy to see Aaron for the first time and spend a few minutes with the boys. When they come in, Aaron crawls toward me, pulls himself up to stand at the couch, lays his head near my knees. He doesn't care how I look. He wants me to hold him but I can't, so I just rub his head for a little while.

"Hi, my sweet Aary," I say, stroking his blond baby hair. "Mommy's back from the hospital! I missed you so much! Did you have a good time at school?"

Noah is chatty about his day. Because of me, his preschool teacher is teaching the kids about doctors and the hospital. The kids are learning about bones and their bodies. "Catch, Mom!" He throws a ball in my direction and I duck, wildly.

Chris groans, reading a notice from Noah's backpack. "Oh man! Apparently there's a pinkeye outbreak!"

Panic rises in my chest. *I. Cannot. Do. This.* Pinkeye? Are you fucking kidding me? No! My poor baby isn't allowed on my lap and Nerf balls are being launched at my busted skull. Now both of my kids could infect my screwed-up eyes.

"I have to go back to the bedroom!" I say loudly.

Once in bed, I sit with my legs crossed under me and *cry*. I go through an entire box of Kleenex, sobbing so hard at one point that I have trouble breathing. This is the closest I've ever come to having a panic attack; it is all too fast, too emotional, too breakable, too unknown. *How am I ever going to get through this?* My right eye has run out of tears. I'm soul weary, destroyed, when Steve knocks to come in.

"How's it going?" he asks, and the tears are back again.

Steve talks to me about being strong, how we have to live life instead of planning it. That, no matter what, we can't predict what's going to happen. He sees me, sees that this is a really extreme version of all that right now, a time when everything's out of my control. Finally, we talk about grief.

My brother describes his own experiences. We rarely get to talk about these things now that we're adults; he's not nearby when I'm having a rough day and I don't often ask for comfort from others, let alone my family. Not since I was a little kid has it worked the other way. But now there's an invitation for just that: another way, a melting down of identity so that it may be reformed, updated. As a young adult I set a secret boundary to never need anyone. Now I cannot do a single thing alone. How many chances do you get for this depth of transformation in one lifetime?

Somewhere, deep down, I wonder if this might be the point. If I was planning the narrative of this life and wanted a way to get me quickly back on track, I might have needed to pull out all the stops. Relearning the ability to ask for help is underneath my entire brain tumor story. Today, family members are living out of suitcases in our living room and parenting my sons. Their efforts are working; we are all okay. It's okay for me to ask them for help.

I have no proof, but it's like the air in the room is receptive to this line of thinking. My angel rep is quiet but feels *present*. I sense that I'm in the right ballpark and I take strength from her support, too.

Eventually, Steve leaves to help with dinner. He will fly home tomorrow, back to my sister-in-law and his job. I miss him already. I close my swollen eyes and I'm still worried, but more calm.

—

"Is your dad out there?" a friend texts. I'm not responding to texts, but if I did I'd say that he's back in New York, that he's a teacher and it's really hard to take time off of school, that he's planning to come next month for a long weekend at Memorial Day. I'm not sure how this sounds. *So you got diagnosed with a brain tumor and your dad didn't even visit?*

That's not how I see it.

My mom recounted telling my dad the news. She said they both sobbed. And once, while waiting for surgery day, I sent my dad an email telling him I loved him. Mom said this made him cry like she had never seen.

I know that our small Berkeley home can only host a certain amount of helpful adults at a time, that many others want to come but we must pace ourselves. My mom is ALL IN being a mom and nurse and nana and mother-in-law. I know that the best thing for my dad is for him to visit when he's ready.

After all, I had wanted Aaron's baby head nestled under my chin so badly that I refused seeing him entirely on my first night home. My options were nothing vs. heart-stainingly-out-of-reach, so I chose nothing. Somehow that was easier.

All of us parent differently when we're struggling to make sense, when we're so close to the edge, when our fragile, human hearts are breaking. I allow love to arrive in whatever form it takes. I don't judge.

CHAPTER 15

MY SECOND NIGHT home is difficult.

Light green dusty curtains are billowing. I can't breathe. I can't escape. I try to get out of this old hospital but there are no exits and as many times as I call for help, nothing comes.

I'm being swung around and around. I try to grab onto the neon-colored plants in the ground, but as I rip them up I see that the leaves all have faces and they are screaming and I'm screaming and they're chasing me.

A moment of quiet. Am I free?

A dusty curtain blows over my head from behind and I realize I'm still in it, I can feel myself going in again, can't breathe, can't get to a friend that I see across the way.

This nightmare is so horrible. I struggle to wake up, aware that it's a dream but clueless as to how to get out of it. When I finally do, I nudge Chris and tell him how scary the dreams are. He rubs my back and tells me I'm safe, that it's not real, but this one is a repetitive dream, coming back again and again, each time even longer and more difficult to escape. Finally around 3am I decide to stay awake for the rest of the night. I ask for help in the dark. Maybe this is a prayer?

Eventually I fall asleep again and dream, but this time everything is different.

———

In this dream, something is unwell inside me.

I'm alone, walking the streets of a familiar city. I know our babysitter is home with the boys, but my time is running out to find an answer for the unrest I feel in my heart. I cannot find help.

I stumble into a party. The music is loud, thick, celebratory.

Men and women move quickly, like elves at the North Pole, up through trap doors and down slides behind the walls. There is an energy of excitement, as if everyone is preparing. Something important is happening here.

I recognize a few faces, men who are well-known. They are the founders and they are joyfully closing this San Francisco office. It hasn't worked out here; they have decided to wrap it up and head back home to New York.

Those running around, preparing for the announcement, are joyous in their relief. "The experiment is over! We are going home!"

Timid to interrupt the scene, but stuck in my own desperate search, I pull one of the founders aside.

"I'm lost," I say. "I'm glad for your happiness but I don't share your story . . ."

"Go see the women," he says, pointing up a level. "They are meeting now and they will be glad to help."

I make my way through the crowded halls and alleyways. A group of beautiful women wearing pastel fabrics are gathered, stunning in their size and presence. Some are packing boxes; all are preparing to go home. Their assignment is over.

One woman is making a necklace whose chain is made of light. Its strands are thin and delicate, yet strong in the way of metal and earthly elements. As she moves it between her fingers, the light shimmers, nearly alive.

From the chain hangs a pale blue number 12.

It is unbelievably beautiful and I want to know where she got it, how she made it, where other things like this are found, but I'm drawn into the scene with the other women.

"We are going home," they celebrate. "We are going home."

I am not like them. I am sad. I am not going home. I don't even know if I have a home.

Inside me, something is unwell. They know my feelings without words. The music still blasts at top volume.

"You are going home too, Jen!" they cheer. "It is over for you, too!"

Could it be, I wonder?!

I open my right eye. The last notes of the loud song still ring in the air. The world is firm again in the way that dreams are not, and when a white strip of fabric comes into focus, I remember:

There is an ice pack on my left eye.

I am recovering from brain surgery.

I was unwell. I had a brain tumor.

But it has been solved.

And now, it is over.

For many minutes I cannot move; the relief is so profound and I don't want to break its beauty. As I lay there, I know that the dream and waking worlds are only separated by a thin veil, that they are both true. My belief is as strong as light.

Outside our window, dawn arrives. Chris breathes next to me; I let him sleep.

I find my phone and clumsily type some lyrics I remember from the dream. What was that song? It was playing so vividly the whole time. Google gives me the answer.

For a Better Day, a song by Avicii.

I'm speechless with the magnitude of this title.

Later this morning, I will tell everyone in the house every detail of the dream. I call it *The Beautiful Dream.* "The women were angels," I say, over and over again. "It is the most beautiful thing I have ever experienced."

And it is! A beautiful scene, a beautiful experience, but most of all a beautiful message. I am no longer unwell. Due to forces larger than I can understand, I have found my way home.

⌒

A few hours later, Mom sets up the stool in the shower. She helps me walk to the bathroom and undresses me, carefully pulling the pajama top over my head. She holds my hands as I step over the side of the tub, then turns on the water once I'm seated. She has helped hundreds of patients in and out of showers but today, she seems anxious. I wonder if she has ever washed someone's fresh head scar.

"Is this too hot?"

"No, that feels nice."

I rub my hand over the back of my head, the tiniest hair fuzz starting to grow. It feels like a baby animal's fur.

The air is cold and I shiver when Mom turns the water off to wash my body. I try not to overthink this moment and make it too sentimental, but it is nice to feel my mom's love so viscerally. When she's done, she helps me step out of the tub again and wraps a big towel around me. It is good to be washed.

I don't need as much help walking back to my room.

⌒

After a nap, I tell my mom that I'm feeling well enough to do something with Noah. Avicii's song from *The Beautiful Dream* is still rolling through my mind, its "better day" message giving me energy.

"Maybe he can help you hang the cranes?" She gathers tape and the pile of paper cranes that grows every time the mail arrives.

"Noah! Your mommy wants to do a special project with you!" I can hear the optimism in her voice. A special project means her daughter is getting better.

Noah, trailed by Chris, comes into the bedroom to find me sitting in the rocking chair, pulling off a couple pieces of tape to attach a crane to our closet door.

"It's okay, we're fine," I say. Chris hesitates, then heads back to the living room.

"Which one should we hang first?" Noah chooses a bright pink crane and presses it onto the door. Next we hang one from my aunt and uncle, then a childhood friend. After a few minutes, my mom leaves the room, too. Holy crap, I'm parenting my boy alone! I take a picture of Noah hanging cranes and, when we're done, I post it on Instagram.

It's May and it hit me last night that I almost didn't see it and that happens now sometimes, a big sadness like that. I don't have any words. I am so so grateful.

For a long time after Noah leaves, I stare at his photo. I rock in the chair, alone, quiet. I barely thought about dying before surgery, but now that things are over and recovery is underway, I'm finally afraid. The tsunami of what could have been crushes me and I sob again without restraint, a mesh of gratitude and terror, a raw heart underneath. I'll be able to do all of the things I love one more time! Trips to favorite cities, dinners with friends, birthdays and anniversaries and ice cream and new books. French. Life is possible again.

My mind is cycling through these cherished possibilities when Muhlenberg's Christmas candlelight service pops into my head. I've attended the service a few times since college, always a nice excuse to go back to Allentown, Pennsylvania, for a nostalgic night and to walk the campus. Muhlenberg's campus is made for memories: lawns and poetic gathering spaces and worn paths where you run into people you know, even years after you've graduated. One day, I will visit it again.

The candlelight service is held in old, stone Egner Chapel. During the service, the choir always begins with an a cappella version of *Once in Royal David's City* and, every time I've attended, chills go through me when their voices join the soloist in the second verse. Hungry to hear it again, I find a version of the hymn on my phone. I play it on repeat and rock in the chair, allowing the loud sound to overwhelm my tender brain.

MRIs. Hospital rooms and medications and beloved friends mailing packages. Our family members waiting for news. My sons—*babies* I'd only just birthed—nearly losing their mother. ICU and lemon loaves and Bay Bridge traffic and my skull sawed open. Somehow, after all this, I am still fucking alive.

Somehow, this is now my life story.

And then it happens. Like a zip file opening in my mind, I know *everything*. For several seconds, in this rocking chair, I understand the universe in each of its possible dimensions.

Everything is real.

Everything is exquisite.

Everything happened: Bible stories, all religions, knights, dinosaurs, faraway lands. It all happened, it is all beautiful and complex and life keeps going in other times and dimensions. It never ends, will never end, our big multi-moving universe.

Nothing is too big.

Nothing is big enough.

These messages are beyond convincing. I sit in awe, afraid to breathe. I replay the song over and over, yearning for more to come, but there will be no more. In the aftermath, a careful, dense peace fills the room.

Like in the MRI vision and while within *The Beautiful Dream*, I know that I will personally survive this crisis, but in the rocking chair messages, I also glimpse something much bigger than we can ever understand. This Bigness is responsible for future visions and life-changing dreams and coincidences, all of it till forever. It makes no sense to dispute others' beliefs because those are also true—we all have access to whatever version of spiritual curriculum we need to navigate our lives, should we reach for it. It is simple and beautiful, this invitation.

I recognize, for the first time, that there's always been a tiny, incessant spot of loneliness in my heart. Through this experience, it is filled.

CHAPTER 16

IN THE DAYS and weeks and months and years that follow those three spiritual moments, I map every angle. Was I on drugs at the time? Absolutely. What would have been the side effects of steroids, vitamins, rash cream, and ibuprofen?

During the episodes, I was: locked in an MRI tube, in a dream following a nightmare, living a grief-filled moment in a rocking chair. None of them arrived at the same time of day or place. During all three events, I was alone. Each time, I wished for the experience to keep going or come again, urging its return by not moving, the way you might stop abruptly when you spot a rabbit up ahead.

Maybe the MRI vision was meant to keep me calm until surgery. Then *The Beautiful Dream* got me to a dreamscape where I could meet my angels in a higher realm. All this so that my gritty sadness and raw gratitude in the rocking chair scratched the veil, causing a tiny rip that let God slip through. Why move so progressively? Why not jump straight to The Bigness?

I don't know. Maybe hearing God's voice directly is simply too much for our fragile, human ears.

From the earliest days of diagnosis, I know that I'm going to write a book. It doesn't feel like an option, rather an inevitability. (Could my angel rep have slipped this assignment to me, too?) I've always wanted to write a book. Now, with a brain tumor, it seems I've found my story.

Throughout these stressful weeks, I send myself emails with the subject line "Book." At all hours of the day, from all sorts of places, I email myself misspelled and meandering notes so that I can remember details about the scenes I'm living through. I use "God" interchangeably with "The Bigness," depending on whether its presence feels powerful or playful in the moment. After the rocking chair experience, I email myself the following:

Subject: Book

I believe in everything

Magic

I believe

I thought the book was going to be a memoir about health and motherhood and finding courage, but now this God stuff has arrived and, with it, an entirely new realm to explore in writing and studying and community and living. God is real! *How about that?*

There is, of course, one rub: It may be bad for business.

No one in the tech industry believes in God, at least not openly. I don't even live in a swing state! Plucky hosts the most soft-skills workshops out there, and now I'm adding a *spiritual memoir* to my repertoire?! But how can I worry about sales funnels when the power of the entire universe is making itself known? In light of such compelling events, logic must take a backseat.

Also, here's something awkward: When the universe proves the existence of God to *you* but not to *your husband*.

While angel reps and dream visions are working overtime in the back bedroom, Chris is being a dad. And a mom. And a son-in-law. And a grateful recipient of the nightly dinner food train. And on and on.

"Hey, can we talk about something?" Chris says as he joins me in our room, having just put the kids to bed. "I'm embarrassed to say this," he says. "Like, it's so strange to even think it."

I'm not sure what's coming. A critique of God?

"I'm watching you go through this terrible time, but also this amazing transformation . . ." he says, and now I know what he's about to say and it is going to sound strange, so I say it for him.

"You're weirdly jealous."

He looks relieved. "I mean . . . yes! A little! How fucked up is that?"

We both laugh because we can't not. Because surgery is over and I'm in healing mode and the beastly tumor has been vanquished.

"Oh, love. Obviously recovery is terrible, but the attention and support and freedom to rest and dream is a fucking gift. I get it."

We're silent for a while. We talk about how we can't answer the "how are you doing?" question anymore. I mean, we try to, but it's impossible to say. Between us, we've switched to asking it differently.

"What feelings are you feeling?" Which is more clunky, but more true.

Tired, sad, hopeful, patient, scared, bored of these days. Stuff like that.

Jennifer Viner said that people my age are hit by the full force of what happened to them about six months later. You get back to physical norms in two to three months, but mentally it takes time to realize what just happened. I'm one week post-op. Six months sounds lifetimes away.

"Listen, I promise that I'm not going to make decisions for

myself that don't mesh with our family's path," I say. "I'm not going to buy land without you."

Chris points out that we're both ambitious rocket ships and he's right. Even in our wedding vows, we talked about how we can do so much more together than we could ever do alone. Plucky Institute and successful memoirs will have to weave themselves into our family's future. We are still on the same page. In reassuring him of this, I reassure myself too, but even after we've turned out the lights, one pesky boundary remains between us: the God stuff. The God stuff will change the way I parent, the way I plan (or not) for the future, the safety net that I see underneath every challenge in our lives from now on.

Chris is snoring. I roll over and recall the Bible stories I learned in church as a kid, the fishermen who were busy reeling in nets when Jesus strolled by. They dropped everything to follow him. This cannot be the story of my faith.

"This is my condition," I say to The Bigness. "My God stuff has to also work with a husband who does not have God stuff. I will pursue you from where I am, without leaving those I love."

The Bigness is amused. The Bigness consents.

Without consulting a pastor or a priest or a rabbi or a shaman or even Google, I begin praying.

Prayer, for me, is clarifying. It's not beating around any bushes, because the whole point is that you're talking to an all-knowing listener, so I drop the niceties and small talk. My prayers name the highest priorities, the loudest emergencies, my biggest hopes and thanks.

Help Chris, I pray. *Let the boys sleep an extra few minutes so Chris can get more rest before the weekend. Let a package come with a new toy to distract the kids for a few minutes when he needs a break. Please. Please.*

Help Mom, I pray. *Help her relax and take a nap, and comfort her as she prepares to go home. Please. Please.*

Help me rest, I pray. *Convince me to lie down even when I don't want to. It helps, it always, always helps. Let Aaron know I love him even though I can't carry him right now. Help us bond in other ways.*

And—if you have an extra second—get the meal train person to bring dessert tonight. Kthxbye.

———

"I'm ready to take a walk alone." My mom thinks this is a great idea, and I promise to stay close. The boardwalk loop around our parking lot is perfect for slow walking within view of the front windows. I slide my shoes on and hold onto the rail carefully as I make my way down the stairs. I open the gate and step away from the yard.

Holy shit. Has someone handed me glitter-filled glasses? Where was this world before surgery? Every flower is a masterpiece, every sprig of rosemary fully realized, with smell and purpose and gift. And it's all just growing here, available for anyone to know! Unreal.

I spy on the birds as I round the first corner, curious about their voices. The trills and chirps are intentional and alive. *How have I heard birds my whole life and never wondered how they got this way?* They are too exquisite to process, too quick and lovely to invent. And the most mind-blowing of all: butterflies. SYMMETRICAL FUCKING BUTTERFLIES. Mirrored wings, patterns and colors and shapes that had to have been invented by artists. I turn the corner of the loop.

Butterflies are real, as are my neighbor's tomato plants and the electric cars that inventive humans dreamed up. I pat the blue USPS mailbox that lets us send letters to loved ones, I wave to curtains keeping shade, I watch the traffic light switch from green to yellow to red, then back again. I love it all. The sun is warm and the day is bright and every single thought that crosses my mind on this walk feels holy.

⸻

Reading and writing is off the table, so much of my time is spent lying quietly. I turn to a gift from a college friend. The Calm Coloring Book is supposed to relax you with a mix of patterns and familiar shapes. Many of the pages are too complex, the lines too thin, that the squinting required makes my forehead and eyes hurt, so I narrow it down to a few pages whose lines are thicker, basic. Like for a child.

I flip through each option, as if planning to order from a menu. Am I hungry for this? Or maybe this? It takes me thirty minutes to choose a picture to color. On this first day, I choose a hummingbird.

My bird is a mix of blues and purples. The leaves around her are various shades of olive, neon green, and brown, but the most dramatic choice I make is that her background is entirely yellow. The vines that hold the leaves are yellow. Even her eye is yellow. It looks like she's flying home from the sun.

As the robins chat outside my window, I close my eyes and wonder: What color should I use for this part of the picture? And easily, naturally, the answer comes to me. Pink. Gray. Brown. Yellow. I let my simplest brain do the choosing, the level at which delight lives.

My mind wanders; sometimes I think about someone or something, but often coloring is entirely mindless work. I imagine my gray matter stretching out into the new void, dancing in the space, freed of that tumor, which had clogged things up for so many years. I spend hours on this first picture, accomplishing the work in tiny increments, even coloring a bit each night before sleep so I can wind down from another long day. Once I've finished, I go over it a second time, pressing the pencils deeper and firmer into the paper to make the boldest impression.

Maybe I will hang the picture in the hallways of Plucky Institute, I think, scratching the date on the bottom when it's finished. *My hummingbird is* beautiful.

CHAPTER 17

I SHARE A photo of me on a short walk, holding Noah's hand, on Facebook.

363 people liked this post.

I scroll through the names. Nancy from Minneapolis. And Kathryn from grad school and shit, there's Scott from elementary school! The comments are even more energizing. A kid who moved away during middle school tells me I have always been so courageous, which makes me reconsider all of my middle school years and the times when I definitely didn't feel courageous. *What do people see in me that I haven't seen in myself?* Every new like and comment adds another dimension.

These messages are overstimulating and I can't do much more than read through and click-like their comments every few days. I haven't responded to texts for weeks. People are helpfully giving me space and I'm not yet ready to break this precious barrier, plus I physically can't do much typing. One afternoon, a wave of emotion when thinking about my friend Leigh sends me over the communication edge.

xo, I text to Leigh. And then I put the phone down.

Within seconds, my phone lights up with her response, a short burst of love via text message. This feels so good, I send the same message to another friend. There's nothing else to say; the updates are on Facebook and the blog. The only thing I want to communicate anymore is love.

—

Chris jumps off the couch.

"I just got an email from one of your clients—apparently they're the agency that built the YouCaring website. They got our story on the front page!"

Money is pouring in—and now, not only from friends and family. Chris shows me the scrolling donation list, $5 and $10 contributions from folks who were moved by our story. My friend Amanda set up the fund to help us with medical bills, babysitters, and plane tickets for family members.

I didn't realize Jen was the Bernie Sanders of brain tumor funds! she texts Chris.

The mail arrives. Among the cards and flowers, there's also a padded envelope whose return address says "Eggers" and it's postmarked from San Francisco. Alarm bells. Inside the envelope is a signed copy of *A Hologram For The King*.

"To Jen! With love and admiration I send you my strength. Dave Eggers."

Uh, how does Dave freaking Eggers know I had a brain tumor?

Then, our regular babysitter forwards us an email from the CEO of Urban Sitter, the service that we used to find her last year.

Hi, this is Lynn, CEO of UrbanSitter. I saw your FB post about Jen Dary. I don't know the family but I was really moved that you posted it and I would love to help them out. I'd love to put a couple hundred dollars in their UrbanSitter account. I'm just going to do it anonymously but wanted to ask you which account

*I should put it in, the mom's or dad's? Keeping my fingers crossed
that all goes well.*

- Lynn

It's like my angel rep has left the generosity burner on high, as if
she forgot to turn off the surprises and gifts once we were already
blown away. *Five stars!* I want to reassure her. *I'm already rating you
five stars!*

Because, if she didn't forget, then what could she possibly need
from me after this? I got to stay alive, I was uplifted and loved by
our community, I have received way more than I ever would have
asked for . . . what's the catch?

"I'm here, I'm listening," I whisper toward the corner of the
room. "What will I owe after all of this grace?"

———

Dreams are so quickly becoming reality that I'm truly unsure what
will happen if I name a desire.

I want the benign news, I pray, leaning my head into Chris's chest
one afternoon. *I just want them to call and tell me that the tumor was
benign and this is truly over. That's all I need.*

A whisper. *Dream bigger.*

I tuck my legs under me, uncomfortable. *Okay then . . . I want to
publish my book.*

Even bigger.

More books after this book.

BIGGER!

I am pushed into the abyss. *OKAY OKAY, interview with Oprah
under her trees! Book made into a movie! This marriage for my whole
life. Strong, healthy, awesome sons. A writing career that spans decades
and cements my words and records the personality behind this busted*

brain so that my great-grandchildren know me. A beautiful plot of land for Plucky Institute with trees and rolling hills and a garden where we grow our food and a pack of dogs that follow me around and space for family to visit and the opportunity to make enormous, beautiful contributions to humans and the world. I WANT IT ALL. Okay?

Silence in response. Finally, finally, it is enough.

———

This morning, the air feels different. Charged. Someone is angry. The familiar sounds of breakfast, changing diapers, showers, come from beyond the bedroom door, but I'm picking up a thick tension in the house, I can almost smell it. After a while, I head out to the kitchen to refill my water bottle. Chris has left to take the kids to daycare and I can see my mom on the front porch. I can tell that she's on the phone with her colleague.

"He's driving me nuts!" she says. I perch on the couch, listening, as she describes her frustrations with Chris. To be fair, she's been sharing 1,000 square feet with us in high-stress conditions for almost two weeks and she leaves tomorrow. It would be weird if she didn't need a release, so I go back to the bedroom to give her some space to vent.

Instead of letting this friction invade, I feel it wash around me, a new sensation. Historically, I stepped into an active role to iron out conflict during tense periods of my childhood, toxic family arguments, and issues between friends, but today I make a different choice. I'm recovering and no one needs me to solve their problems. Instead, I text Kate.

Me: Hey—Mom is frustrated with Chris. I think they need some space. Can you help?

Kate: On it. I'll take her shopping for baby clothes.

Such is the value of siblings. Mom has been taking care of everyone else for weeks and won't ask for a break or a nap or a shopping trip for her upcoming grandchild. In response, we've learned how to anticipate Mom's needs when she's far too proud to ask for help.

I used to return home from college, from Paris, for the weekend or for a year to save money on rent, and it was the same every time. My role involved grabbing a bucket and emotionally hosing down my family, keeping my own needs to a minimum to account for their stress. No one asked me to take on this responsibility, but there are some jobs in life that you apply for and others that you just start doing. Brain surgery is showing me what it would look like to be different in my family system. I haven't been this forgiving in a long time.

Chris comes home later in the afternoon with two Mother's Day gifts. First, he hands Mom a set of colored pencils and a coloring book.

"Maybe this will help you destress on all the plane rides you take for Genentech," he says. Mom is touched and teary; the shopping break with Kate has given her some breathing room and she's already missing us. I can't imagine what it must be like to see your daughter—fully grown, self-sufficient, and raising her own family—with her life in peril.

Now it's my turn. Chris's hands are shaking as he hands me a square gray jewelry box. I open the lid and find a gold necklace strung with tiny light blue sapphires. The color is exactly like in *The Beautiful Dream* and I cover my face with my hands, already crying.

"Count them," Chris says, crying hard.

"No!" Sure enough, there are twelve.

"The day after you told me about the dream, I went to the jewelry store on 4th Street. I told them what I needed and they made it work; they made this especially for you."

I obviously can't speak. My mom is crying too; she steps toward the door.

"I'm going to give you guys a few minutes."

In the movie version of this scene, it cuts away at some point and fades into the next day, but living it doesn't allow us to skip through time. We hold each other for a while, first sobbing, then sniffling, then just quiet. Chris gets up to make coffee. I gaze at my twelve sapphires. Eventually I take the necklace back to the bedroom and put it on the shelf of my nightstand, on top of books and next to colored pencils, inches away from the spot where I dreamt it in the first place.

⁓

Our meal train delivery is late. I'm mad but also grateful to be alive and I haven't yet figured out how to be both.

"It should be here soon," Mom says.

I deeply feel everyone's energy. It collects in me and though I've been hands-off others' happiness levels for weeks, I'm bordering on physically functional. I huff in my seat at the dinner table, where I've set myself up to wait, no longer a pitiful patient. Now I can tell that I'm actively annoying people.

Dinner arrives, taco salad, which is difficult for me to eat through one side of my mouth. *Who orders taco salad for a person with a detached temporalis muscle?* As Chris gathers the kids to the table, I start eating without them. My head low to the plate, I shovel bits of chicken, lettuce, tomatoes, cheese, and sharp-edged tortilla chips into the right side of my mouth. Half of it falls back out, but so what? My fingers grab the fallen pieces, cram them back in.

By this point, Mom and Chris have taken their seats at the table with the boys, but I can't look at them because I know I'll laugh at the way they're pretending I'm not a hurricane of taco salad. I'm not yet ready to release my pride, and they're still too careful with me to call me out. It isn't until weeks later when Mom's back for another visit when I bring it up.

"Remember the day I ate taco salad like a legit *hog*?" And all three of us are instantly in hysterics, tears sweeping down our cheeks, the veil of recovery's politeness lifted.

CHAPTER 18

MOM IS GONE and reinforcements have arrived: Chris's dad, Kim, and his stepmom, Beth. We are so tired that we don't even know what to ask of them. Finding the tumor and brain surgery were hell, but post-surgery has settled in and I now see that recovery with small kids is the real war. We expend all our energy, attempt to recharge, then do it all again.

Though many family members have offered to come and help, we've invited Kim and Beth because they're a two-person team and can handle two very young boys without us. This opens up new possibilities for Chris to rest. He books a night at an Airbnb nearby so he can relax, watch TV, and get a full night of sleep. On the way out, Chris hands his dad the keys to the rental car. He reshares the address of the kids' daycare and points out the stack of handwritten instructions that my mom left. Lucky for us, Kim is also a nurse.

Chris slings his backpack over his shoulder, obviously nervous to leave. "Go! Go! We'll be fine here," Kim says, and I wave in agreement. The grandparents have raised sons; they will figure out where the bath towels are and what the kids will (or will not) eat. The boys will get over their shyness with the new visitors quickly, and even if they don't, this is where we are.

—

Beth is folding Aaron's clean onesies. Chris, back from his night away, is lying on the couch and Kim is next to him, watching TV. Extended family visits like these are usually packed with trips to the zoo or local tourist attractions, but today the house feels casual and domestic. When would we have ever had these slow moments with Kim and Beth, if not for an emergency? I'm grateful.

The mail will arrive after lunch. I'm worried about the arrival of one particular package, a deck of tarot cards that I stealthily ordered from Amazon last night. One of my favorite bloggers teaches an online tarot class several times a year, and I've always been curious but reluctant to try. Last night, I decided I was finally ready to check it out.

And though *I* may be ready for tarot mysticism, I'm embarrassed for my in-laws to know. Hell, I don't even want Chris to see the deck. I don't know how much more patience others have for my spiritual journey before they assume I've gone from woo-woo enlightened to plain Jane bonkers.

—

"I want to play with Aaron for a few minutes, by myself." The grandparents smile encouragingly.

"Maybe you can play with him while we get dinner ready?" Chris says.

I settle myself in the boys' bedroom with a few toys: a small train, a few ABC blocks, a stuffed bear. Nothing that lights up or makes noise.

"Come on, Aariboo Caribou," Chris says. "Mommy wants to play with you."

He sets Aaron on the carpet and turns to me.

"Want me to leave the door open?"

I shake my head. My baby and I are closed in together.

I decide to reserve my energy by not speaking, driving the train across my lap to Aaron's legs. He pats my hand and I let him have the toy. I show him the wheels, how they turn. Firmly grasping, he bangs the train on the floor. I let him play however he likes for a few minutes until he gets bored.

Next I hand him the blocks, stacking two and offering him the third. He claps. We play like this for a few minutes, focused solely on three blocks. Then I wiggle the stuffed bear against his belly and he laughs. I still haven't said a word, but I touch his back while he crawls around me. Our play is very simple.

We hear someone moving plates around in the kitchen, setting up for dinner. Noah is outside the door and he wants to know what we're doing. I look at my phone. We've been playing for eleven minutes! What a stretch! Chris knocks and says that the dinner has been delivered. Are we ready to eat?

"You can take him," I say quietly, heading back to our room. "It was good, but I'm wiped."

I need an hour in bed with my eyes closed to recover. Still, this is progress.

———

Noah's teacher invites me and Beth to join the class for snack since we missed the Mother's Day celebration last week. This sounds like a good first outing. I can only handle preschool-level conversation and I'm hiding from adults who will want updates. I'm anxious about my scarred, shaved head, but I wear a large floppy hat gifted by a friend. Sure enough, when Noah's teacher greets me in the lobby, she hugs me and cries hard. I look so different.

Once in the classroom, we sit at the table among the three-year-olds. God, it's all so familiar. Cubbies with tiny backpacks, water bottles, packed lunches, lost sweatshirts, and extra shoes.

"This is your hat?" says a boy.

"Why your hair is like that?" a girl asks.

I nod and say this is my new hat, yes, I had a haircut, yes, I'm still Noah's mama. Soon the kids are more interested in their apple slices than my head, and their chatter turns to TV shows and the different animals they saw at the zoo. We only stay twenty minutes, but it's good and I can tell that Noah is proud to have me there, weird headgear and all. He stays very close, only moving off my lap once to get more snack.

———

I don't remember the moment when we learned that my tumor was benign, but the news came quietly through a message on the patient portal. I was on the couch or in bed or at the kitchen table, and Chris or Beth or Kim or the boys were there or they were not. It was morning or afternoon or it was evening and it was sunny. Or it was not. The details of the scene have been lost to me.

Whatever words the pathologists used, this is what I heard: *Your life has been renewed.*

Beyond exquisite, a second chance, my priceless wish granted.

CHAPTER 19

THREE WEEKS POST-OP, we're back at UCSF. I've been worried that getting stitches out would hurt, but I didn't need to; Jennifer Viner has a steady, easy hand.

"What are you taking for pain?" she asks as she snips.

"Advil, but not that often." I tell her I stopped the narcotic within a day of being home.

"The scar doesn't hurt," I say. "But I can't believe how little I can do."

She wheels the black stool over to her desk, makes a note.

"Recovery is slow and fast," she says. "You're on the right track."

She prepares to send us on our way, to return in three weeks for the final checkup with McDermott.

"Then what happens?" I ask.

"Then you'll come back in a year," she says, sliding her paperwork into a bright blue folder.

Chinese food at the Panda Express is hard to resist and I'm not rushed to leave, so we stop in the cafeteria for lunch. I catch my reflection in the glass windows; my face is still round, chubby, swollen. Ew.

BE ADVENTURESOME, says my fortune cookie. TRY A NEW LOOK.

"I'm really nailing this one," I say, showing the slip to Chris. He laughs.

For a month, the whiteboard has been propped up against our closet door. The names of brain surgeons, their phone numbers, and the hospitals they work at are scrawled across it in my own shocked handwriting. To erase it would be significant, like admitting that we are finally past that day, as if I'm starting to move on.

I can see the whiteboard from bed, where I'm coloring. I focus on my pencil strokes—this image has small circles inside flowers. The detail is challenging my vision so I can only color one at a time, taking short breaks by forcing my eyes elsewhere in the room. Eventually I push the blankets off my legs and move myself carefully to the floor, where I crawl over to the board. I stare at it again for a few minutes, holding my palm up against my handwritten marks.

I am not rushed. I realize that I could spend all afternoon with my hand on this whiteboard, saying goodbye to the scariest day of my life. I have no meetings to get to, my business is closed, and other people are taking care of my kids. I could decide to sit here every day for a week, for a month even, if I needed. To be present with this grief, to befriend it, to watch it calm itself down, is magical. I can feel my breath and the beat of my heart. I imagine grabbing the eraser, noting my body's reaction, a muscular clench. *What will I replace this with?* I wonder. And then I know: I will write a list of goals.

Today or next week or next year, the only way I can replace these brain surgeon names is with a list of recovery goals. My body reacts differently to this idea. *We know how to do goals!* my muscles hum.

I'm thinking about which goals I might consider when my

thumb strokes the board, accidentally erasing part of McDermott's name—oops!—and my body tenses up again. I reach for my phone to snap a shot before the memory of this board is lost, and now that I've documented it, my body is calm again. I sit with my palm flat against the board, as if I'm at a gravestone, remembering my past self. I wait until the grief is fulfilled and I am bored.

No one lives in cemeteries, I think. *At some point you have to go home.*

With large, sweeping movements, I wipe the whole board clean. Fresh. I uncap the green marker. In careful, childlike handwriting, I form the letters: *G O A L S.* Then I make a list.

- pick up Aaron
- make pancakes
- walk in Tilden Park
- visit Kate's chickens
- go to Paper Source
- write a letter
- drink wine
- watch kids alone
- watch *House of Cards* final episode
- cross stitch
- go to a coffee shop alone
- go to any church
- write Anthony (4/8 MRI tech) a note

Some of these sound impossible. If I can't make it through ten minutes of *Seinfeld,* how will an hour of *House of Cards* go? Watching the kids alone will require lifting the damn baby. Stitching even a small Christmas ornament feels eons away.

But I've been able to do more every day so far and these goals don't have a deadline. Still, I challenge myself to walk to Paper Source by the end of the week.

—

Two days later, *Make pancakes:* CHECK.

A chore that normally takes fifteen minutes consumes more than an hour; the house is filled with smoke by the time we eat, but I get it done!

Things I'm more patient about now: not getting every last drop from the bowl, batter splatter on the counter, waiting for an egg to separate.

—

Chris is spending another night at an Airbnb and I'm having a nightmare. When I wake up, my heart is pounding and I'm alone in our bed. I stay awake in the dark until Aaron cries at 5:15. I have just been cleared to lift him (CHECK!) so I carry him into the living room, where Kim and Beth are having early coffee on the couch. Beth wraps a knit blanket around my shoulders and rubs my back while I cry and recount the dream. Kim sits with Aaron on the floor. It could be awkward, crying to my in-laws, but recovery is dropping walls, leaving me bare and open to welcome another kind of parenting.

I'm reminded of my semester abroad at college, when I lived with a host family in Aix-en-Provence who had four children and a big fat cat named Basil. My host parents, Janick and Gérard, treated me like one of the family. Though I was older and taller than my host siblings, I was about as useless as the toddler in many situations, especially those that required fluent French.

My own parents were going through a difficult period while I was abroad. It was the school year that started with 9/11—the world was falling apart and I didn't have anyone to talk to about it, not about the attacks or about my parents. Limited to baby French, I kept a lot of my feelings inside.

One night, Janick made me cocoa after dinner. The kids were watching TV in their rooms and she sat across from me at the table in flowered cotton pajamas.

"Now, Jennifer," she said. "What is it? What is in your heart?"

I cried. Not about 9/11, which had happened mere weeks earlier and was too traumatic and absurd to process yet, but about my family, my parents, feeling far away from my siblings, the responsibility I felt to keep them all at peace. How hard it was to decide when to leave and live my own life, when the duty of daughter and sister called me to stay! Janick came around the table and held me, her soft pajamas warm against my face.

"Now," she said. "Jennifer, this is not for you to be troubled about. Your parents want you to be strong and grow free. They will work it out."

I thought she was entirely wrong. I didn't have confidence that they would work it out, and I was not convinced that they understood how to let me grow free. Janick had never seen how much my mom sobbed every time I left for college. But Janick was a mother too, the only other kind of mother I'd had so far. A *host* mother. Through her, I experienced the unique intimacy of being parented by others, supplementing—but not replacing—my own parents.

When Noah wakes around six, Beth encourages me to lie down again. I walk the hallway, sleepiness creeping in, keeping the blanket wrapped around me even as I tuck myself into bed.

⌒

And could I think of God as another kind of parent? This is what I'm imagining when I wake up. Of course there's the Christian perspective, that God is a father, but as I mull it over, I'm not sure I need another parent. I might, however, really like an extra *grandparent.*

What I remember most about all of my grandparents is this: I did not hold any responsibility. On both sides, my grandparents were always just happy to see me, curious to ask a little about my life and game for me to ask them questions. It was a very simple relationship.

So what if I thought of Bigness as a grandparent? Grandma God? An elder, wise and warm, familiar as a pilled sweater, someone who cared about and rooted for me and, no matter what, told me everything would be all right. I spend the next hour imagining this Grandma God. When I'm frustrated with the limitations of recovery, I lie back on the pillow and pretend I'm leaning into her lap. When I can tell everyone in the house is tired of each other, I feel her behind me.

This is not yours to worry about, Grandma God whispers calmly. *This is their work. You're safe here with me.*

CHAPTER 20

FIVE WEEKS POST-OP. Kim and Beth have gone home to Wisconsin and I'll be taking over kid duty next week when Chris returns to work. He and the boys have just returned from the library and Noah is telling his first lie.

"Mommy said I could have a treat after I went to the library."

"Are you sure?"

"Yes," says Noah.

"Let's go check in with her." I hear them coming down the hallway, a gentle knock at the door, then they arrive at the foot of the bed.

"Are you still napping?" Chris asks. I shake my head.

Noah trails Chris, his head down. Before Chris even says a word, he bursts into tears; his jig is up.

"Come here, buddy," I say, sitting up and inviting him to my side of the bed. I hate that he is feeling shame in his little three-year-old self. He climbs onto my lap and I reassure him that he can just ask for a treat if he wants one, he doesn't have to make it up. He is sniffling now, nodding; he understands.

These little hands, my baby! This thoughtful little boy who is mine, who has been such a sidekick these past weeks. Never a burden, always one of my two reminders of why it's so important to keep healing.

I want to raise him. I want to see him and his brother through their lives. I ask Chris to close the door and I rage with bottomless grief for an hour. It is all too much. It is too overwhelming to ask me to parent my kids while I am handling this *mindfuck*.

I avoid the Eleanor Roosevelt sign with my eyes and purposefully avoid looking at cranes or anything inspiring in my room. Fuck it all! Poor sweet Noah, lying about cookies, visitors coming and going and never knowing who would pick him up at the end of each school day! How dare this happen to him, to me! How dare I build a life that I was proud of only to land in this shitstorm, to watch my children and husband struggle like this!

I descend into fury. Not *one* of my habits are the same in this new life. I'm playing with tarot cards! I'm coloring for hours with colored fucking pencils. I'm eating cheese sticks at 3am and receiving greeting cards and books in the mail from favorite authors. Now God is in the picture, too. It has been too beautiful to have ever imagined—but all this is ugly, ugly, ugly too.

I haven't done bedtime with my sons alone in over a month. I had to close my beloved business, the one that I was working so hard to grow. I can't listen to music or read or drive and who knows when I will travel again. My husband is holding this all together. This story—MY story—is a constant weight on all our shoulders.

My head is FAT and UGLY.

Whose life is this?

I cry and cry. I use all the Kleenex. My eyes are puffy, especially the left one.

I skip dinner and lay alone for a while, eyes closed. Then I send a message to a friend who was sick with cancer last year; now she's in remission and she's frank about low points. It's good to hear about someone else's bad. Evening moves into night. Eventually, the energy of grief passes.

During my final checkup, McDermott says that 50 percent of meningiomas recur within 25 years. Maybe, to some, this sounds reassuring, but it breaks my heart. Chris later explains that, because mine was Simpson Grade 1, reoccurrence is much less likely, but still. I cannot stand the idea of going through this again.

I'm able to read more now. In fact, I reread the first Harry Potter, get through the second, and am into the third book by the time my parents visit over Memorial Day. It really pisses me off that Voldemort shows up in each book and when Harry narrowly defeats him, no one says, "LET'S JUST FINISH HIM OFF FOR GOOD." The guy is weak but he still exists.

And yet. I also think about how Harry kicks it in third year, hanging with friends and learning lots and having a fun time on a broomstick, all while knowing evil Voldemort is still out there, waiting. Harry doesn't let it hold him back. He doesn't let it keep him down.

Six weeks post-op, Chris is back at work and I am alone all day. I publish this essay on Medium:

Identity

I. One of the packages waiting for me when I got home from the hospital was from Stitch Fix. In the whirlwind of events leading up to brain surgery, I'd forgotten to postpone or even cancel the service that I rarely used and had lukewarm feelings about. I arrived home with a swollen, purple face and a bloody head; it was not my most empowering fashion moment and as my husband helped me back to our bed, I figured we would just send it back without opening it.

The next morning, however, the kids went off to daycare and I asked my mom if she could help me try on some of the clothes. A flowered tank top was at the top of the box; I put it on and grimaced. *Not really my style,* I thought. But then I confronted my first identity challenge.

What WAS my style?

When everything you know to be true about your life is suddenly shaken to the very core, it's hard to pin logic and predictions on just about anything. *Were* we done having children? Was I even going to be around to raise the two we had? As my loving husband helped me and the kids through the longest and most intense days of our lives, I often felt like we needed to start back at a first date to re-meet each other. Because even "Are you religious?" had become a question that I answered differently post-surgery.

So there I am, staring at myself in the mirror wearing a floral tank top, and I just decided then and there: Flowers are beautiful. They're alive. They are definitely my style.

I kept the shirt.

II. My maiden name is Epting. When Chris and I got engaged and discussed whose names were becoming what, one option on the table was to combine Epting and Dary and become the Darings. (I KNOW.) We dropped the idea and I took his name but, riding high on surviving brain surgery and hearing the tumor was benign, I brought it up again one night before bed.

"Okay, totally unrelated topic: *Should* we change our names to the Darings?!" Chris started laughing. He was exhausted and so was I, but we talked it out, ultimately dropping it again.

Would it have been a crazy thing to do? Yep. Would it have involved 1,000 pounds of paperwork and DMV misery and new birth certificates and awfully confused in-laws? You bet. But if we had felt up for it, I would have done it all. I would have owned the cheesiness and ridiculousness and looked forward to a time when I'd be called up to give a talk at a conference as "Jen Daring." Because when you evolve and grow, nothing is pinned down or unchangeable—even your name.

III. I have a buzz cut and a big scar and now people recognize me. The baristas at the coffee shop I frequented a few times a week have only now started remembering my order. What do they think happened? Is it obvious that I had brain surgery? I'm usually good at seeing the world from others' eyes, but this is a huge blind spot for me now. I simultaneously want to tell the story and avoid telling it ever again.

I made a new friend the other day, a fellow mom at the boys' daycare. We got coffee. She doesn't compare me with what I used to look like; she can't answer the question "Do I seem like myself?" because my current self is as authentic as she expects it to be. Sometimes I get so involved in the conversation and then go to the bathroom only to be shocked in the mirror as I wash my hands. *Has she been staring at this head the whole time we've been talking?*

It is so strange.

It is so so strange.

IV. I have been struggling with owning my feminine identity since the surgery. Though my buzz cut is growing out, there is a large hairless scar across the middle of my head and it will be a while before I re-find wavy tresses. In an industry with many men and as a mom to two boys, I used to exert my femininity just by existing. I wore jeans and Toms and simple gold hoop earrings and still felt like a woman.

I guess it's the loss of my hair, but now my feminine self feels cloudy.

Probably as a reaction to this, I chose bright pink nail polish for a pedicure recently, the opposite of what I used to get, which was clear. But, as with the flower shirt, it didn't feel like a betrayal of self or style to mess with bright pink; my identity has been busted wide open and all choices seem possible.

There is a rich space between nature and nurture, between self and momentum. Who are you? And who are you because you've inherited a label or choice or style, even if you were the one who originally chose it?

I feel gratitude to have this space of half-baked identity after a huge life event. At thirty-five years old, I'm experiencing a rebirth in which I can change almost anything that needs an update in my identity. But what does one do if she doesn't have a disruption in her life? How do you give yourself permission to change, to break the momentum of what others believe to be your role or identity?

Well, I'll give it to you. Here is your permission slip to change something fundamental because you have outgrown what was there before. Get a bike and start riding it everywhere. Chop off your hair (or let it grow long!). Tell your family you don't want gift cards anymore to the stores you loved in 2005. Pull your manager aside and tell her that the skills you were hired for aren't the only tools in your toolbox. Buy a deck of tarot cards, plan a solo vacation, bravely email someone you deeply admire and see if they write back.

Because you are allowed to change without a brain tumor

to justify it. You are allowed to find new versions of yourself so your identity continues to authenticate; it doesn't make you a betrayal to what was.

It makes you an adult who is growing and evolving and maturing. And damn, if we don't need more of these kinds of humans to help run our world.

Two weeks after I post the essay, there's another package in the mail. I'm on my way to yoga, so I throw it in the car and open it while I wait for the studio to open.

To: Jen Daring :)

From: Your Stitch Fix family

Inside are two custom mugs. Inscribed on each is a name: Mr. Daring, Mrs. Daring. I cry against the steering wheel.

Imagine! Some person at Stitch Fix read my story on Medium. This person was moved. This person took action, maybe asking a boss for budget or maybe paying for it herself. This person saw a way to contribute to my story, generously, relatively anonymously, with grace.

Mr. Daring is at work when I text him an image of our new mugs.

I believe in humans. I believe in humans. I believe in humans.

I hold this phrase throughout my whole yoga class, moving my own human body to the teacher's instructions. At the end of class, I lay on my back in Savasana, teary and more than a little grateful.

⌣

After yoga, I always head to the coffee shop next door, where I read and write. I'm trying to maintain some sort of schedule while the boys are at daycare. I have been to the library to see what books they have about recurring tumors and googled support groups and resources for meningiomas. There are (rightly so) tons of resources for cancer survivors. But there's not much for someone whose tumor was benign.

Today, I order coffee and toast. I pull out my latest library books: one about Buddhism, one about medical miracles, and one called *Radical Remission: Surviving Cancer Against All Odds*. I am three bites into my toast when I realize what this looks like.

I have no hair.

I have a large scar across my head.

I am flipping through a book about surviving cancer.

Quickly, I hide the book in my bag. What if someone assumes I am a cancer survivor? That pity is not mine to claim. That support or prayer should go toward someone who's in worse shape, whose diagnosis was malignant.

Should I switch to a Kindle? Make a book cover out of a brown bag like we used to do in middle school? Hold up a sign: *Feel bad for me but not too bad?* I don't pull the book out again. Instead, I finish the toast and open my laptop to make notes for my own book.

And this is exactly the spot I'm in, same table, two days later when I meet Levi Felix for the first time.

CHAPTER 21

I'M WEARING HEADPHONES and looking at my screen when I notice a man trying to get my attention. He's waving. I take out my earbuds.

"Excuse me, did you have a craniotomy?"

I am taken aback.

"Because I did," he says. His hair is pretty short and I can see the hint of a rainbow scar across his head. He tells me that his craniotomy was in February. His hair is two months longer than mine.

"Who did your surgery?" he asks.

"Michael McDermott at UCSF Parnassus." His face lights up.

"He was my surgeon too!"

I joke that we should start a local branch of the McDermott alumni; also maybe Levi should adopt my nickname for our favorite, best neurosurgeon: McDrizz.

"Wait, who's your oncologist?" Ah. Right.

"Oh," I say. "Actually, I was really lucky. My tumor was a meningioma. It was benign."

To his credit, Levi doesn't break stride.

"Oh, I have a GBM. That's why I haven't seen you at support group."

"No," I say quietly. "I haven't found . . . I mean. Yeah. I didn't know about that group."

GBM means glioblastoma, the most aggressive form of brain cancer out there. That's the one my mom feared most.

Levi doesn't live in Berkeley; he's just up here sometimes for treatments in San Francisco. His fiancée, Brooke, is living with him at his parents' house and she's helping him get around. Right now she's at the grocery store across the street. We exchange information and agree to have coffee the next time they're in town.

When we meet up two weeks later, Brooke joins us.

Levi is a little younger than me; he's thirty-two. He cofounded an organization with Brooke called Digital Detox, an adult summer camp designed to help people relax without devices. We talk about this for a while and then I tell them about Plucky.

"Oh! Any interest in acquiring DD?" he asks, mostly joking, but also maybe a little not.

I smile and say that Plucky is paused for a while. I tell him a little bit about Plucky Institute, skirting most of the spiritual parts. Levi is a fan of being outside and learning from each other; maybe Plucky Institute and DD can partner one day.

We switch topics to his new meal plan. Brooke knows most of the details; Levi leans back, quiet. I recognize well this need to rest, so I focus on Brooke. She tells me how he's been handling the most recent treatments, how sometimes he's confused or forgetful. Levi smiles and makes a joke about their dynamic. They are like an old married couple—Levi relying on Brooke, who is tracking his medication doses and creating meal plans that sound like hell to keep up. Brooke outlines some of the future surgeries he'll need as things progress with his tumor and I take all of this in, politely, as if Brooke and I have more in common—because despite my and Levi's matching head scars, maybe it's true. Only one of us here has brain cancer.

They talk a little about wedding planning. Levi lightly mentions having children, maybe moving to a farm and getting goats. Living simpler. He has clearly redrawn the district lines for his life. I walk home from our coffee, emotionally destroyed. Chris is at work and the kids are at daycare and the downstairs neighbor is at school so I make sure the windows are closed and then I scream.

"*WHY ME?*" I yell toward the ceiling. "WHY WASN'T THAT ME? WHY WAS I SO LUCKY? WHAT DO YOU WANT FROM ME?"

I stalk the room, hurling pillows, throwing my entire body at the immoveable couch to feel its resistance over and over, three times, four times, feral.

Sweet Levi! He has a FIANCÉE, you know! He wants to be a dad! He is making this world better! He takes people to the fucking woods and plays his guitar for them so they can live better lives! Why was HIS cancer? Why is HE at the support group? Why am I HERE?

If guilt and gratitude and anger and luck had a baby, it would be me. I don't see a fucking point to anything. These life minutes pass, adding up to hours, nine-to-five jobs, then two days off on the weekends if you're lucky. Life life life life, three meals a day, unrelenting life. So many people sleepwalk through it, ignorant of the absurd ease they take for granted.

Today, I give no benefits of the doubt. I am not generous with my metaphors—in fact, metaphors are ugly. Because Levi has brain cancer and I do not. Literally.

Meeting Levi nine weeks post-op pushes me to a complex place. I come into a constant tug-of-war between my abilities and my desires and my euphoric state fades as life returns to a somewhat normal rhythm. I feel lonely, lost, untethered from any true north. What comes after recovery? No one has ever told me.

As life starts to reassemble, pre-surgery life and regular responsibilities are shifting back to my plate and I'm losing God. There was no space for her before and so there is nothing carved out to slide back into. Will I go *back* to my life or will I go *forward* to my life? It is completely my choice.

One morning, I'm at a café with the boys when a dad comes in with two young kids and we start talking about parenting. He says that he'd read an interesting article the other day in which the writer suggested that we have experiences over and over until we learn how to move past them. I say that I've heard something similar in my travels. The kids are passing around grimy blocks. Something clicks.

After I gave birth to Aaron, I'd had the opportunity to come back to work slowly but I rushed into a frenetic schedule, burning out again within a few months. I could have saved some space to write or to see friends or to exercise or even to just sleep, but I didn't want someone to say I wasn't hungry enough for the business, not mothering enough to be a mom, so I stepped back into it all, full-force.

Also: I've run Plucky for others' approval from the beginning, afraid of claiming all the benefits of being a business owner. I haven't even given myself vacation days! I would never work for a company this disrespectful to its employees if it were not my own. Furthermore, I have ideas for a management training, essays to write, coaching services to add, but I haven't been brave enough to try them. I've been afraid of what everyone would think, this girl who studied French and now is trying to boldly insert herself into a digital industry that belongs to others.

Where is my self-respect? Why am I waiting for everyone else to approve my life?

After everything that's happened in the past year, I see that I am my only limit. Building this kind of life could be a team effort; I've got a whole new support system in The Bigness and Grandma God and my angel rep and dreams and mystical unseen energies, silence and nature and creativity and gratitude. *Am I ready to live?*

The answer arrives, quiet as thirst. I choose the road marked *forward.* I make some space for God.

PART III

CHAPTER 22

I WOULD NEVER say it out loud, but I now believe I'm invincible. The Bad Thing has happened and I've accepted the Divine, so I move into a season of risks and infinite rewards. My trust in greater things secures me a flawless safety net. This is what I believe.

The Bigness has found me in my bedroom, an MRI machine, a hospital . . . where can I regularly find her? One assumes church could help with that. I'm driving the boys up to Tilden Park when we pass it, All Souls Episcopal Church of Berkeley. The exterior is simple: gabled roofs, natural materials, no steeple, but I'm leery of the word *Episcopal*. Isn't that the fanatical, judgmental megachurch? I look it up later and find that *Episcopal* is not the word *Evangelical*, just different "E" denominations. The Episcopal Church is known for its social justice work. Interesting.

The 2016 presidential election is eight weeks away when I visit All Souls for the first time. Not wanting to test a religious atmosphere with everyone, I only bring Noah. The inside of the church is lined with colorful stained glass windows and filled with wooden pews and interesting art. You get the feeling you could spend a long time alone in this sanctuary, exploring all of the intentional spaces tucked away for prayer.

Along the back wall is a large statement: *All Souls Are Mine*

Saith The Lord. Noah and I sit toward the back on a large carpet laid out with toys and I settle into the opening hymn, surveying the bulletin while we sing. There's a lot going on at this church: adult classes, social outings, multiple services per week. When the rector asks if there are any new people today, I keep my head down, pretending that Noah needs me. I don't like the public nature of those kinds of introductions because I feel pressure to justify why I'm there and, today, I want to be an observer.

During the sermon, the rector connects a recent trip to the grocery store with the Gospel. In unpacking the Greek word for *forgiveness*, he jokes that half the congregation could probably translate it better than him. Apparently I'm among clever linguists and UC Berkeley professors. Cool.

While her colleague preaches, the associate rector nurses her son in the front row. Wait. There's a female priest? She's a mom? She's nursing her baby under her robes? This is more modern than I've ever imagined church to be.

After the service, Noah and I walk downstairs to the summer children's class, where the kids are making stained glassed windows with colored cellophane. The nursing priest, Liz, is there with her older daughter, who is about Noah's age. I confide that it's our first time visiting All Souls and Liz is kind and measured with her welcome. She isn't pushy, she doesn't say "Jesus" all the time, and she seems like a cool mom who also happens to believe in God. I mean, she has made The Bigness her *career*.

I like All Souls enough to return, not every week but often, particularly while seeking comfort after the election results. I feel held in a sort of curriculum, a spiritual school where we're processing worldly events together.

One day Liz preaches about losing her second child when he was four weeks old. I haven't heard this story before and it catches me unaware; Liz has trauma, too. We're all glued to the pews, hanging on Liz's framing, the details of such a deep tragedy. Liz is going before us, modeling what it's like to hold horrible stories against The Bigness—and not to run off. I imagine how easy it would have been for her to turn away from her faith; how can you be a foot soldier for God when it took your child? This level of authentic complexity is what I'm here for. All Souls is an entire room, building even, of people saying real things.

Finding God in community is a new layer to my faith. I'm still defining what I believe and it's hard to fit these experiences into one entirely well-organized historic religion, so I don't. I never pray to Jesus; I generally don't think about him. Other parishioners wear crosses around their necks and we say his name all the time during service, but Jesus feels like grad school, while I'm still back in elementary school with The Bigness. I'm such a baby in my faith that I need a presence whose skirt I can hide behind, something as simple as nature and stars and closing my eyes and focusing on my breath. Jesus and his story requires a lot more heavy lifting. Son of God? Born to a virgin? Died and then got undead three days later? Hard to embrace.

I steer clear of services that last until midnight and involve dunking grown adults in a large bathtub because I met The Bigness when I was all alone, its shape my perfect complement. I find it hard to experience cosmic intimacy in a public setting, but I do love the weekly structure of tradition and community and making new friends who are also interested in whatever else is out there.

⌒

Nine months post-op. A woman is defending herself from a man who is choking her so I move off the mat to make more room. The self-defense instructors switch roles to show the maneuver again and I'm questioning my choice of this Friday night activity. We're only thirty minutes into class when a song starts repeating between my ears. A cross between a thought and a memory, I can *feel* the song, the rhythm of its lyrics, but I can't access the words. *What song is this?* And why am I distracted by a random song, when I might be paying attention to the feisty classmate trying to pin me to the ground? I excuse myself and go into the bathroom, where the tune remains trapped on replay.

What

is

happening?

I'm not nauseous or faint—it's just that my train of thought is stuck on this song. I splash my face with cold water and look in the mirror. Is this dangerous? Come on. It's a song. Aware that I'm hogging the bathroom, I pour myself a glass of water in the lobby, where the teacher finds me. She read my medical history on the registration form when I entered the gym an hour earlier.

"Everything okay?"

Oddly, my vocabulary is limited to the most basic words.

"I'm not sure," I say. "I think I need to go."

She asks if I'm okay to drive and I understand her question. My comprehension isn't affected.

"I'll stay in the car," I say. "When I'm okay, I'll go."

Winter in Northern California is never cold, but it's chilly enough that I turn the car on for the heat and sit for ten minutes, then ten more. Eventually pride overcomes caution and I drive the 0.9 miles home. Chris and I assume I should have had more water; maybe I didn't eat enough dinner before class; also I'm about to get my period; maybe it's even some craniotomy side effect. These things happen, right? I take two Advil and go to bed.

During this first year post-op, two other auditory-related events occur. Once, as I'm giving bedtime instructions to a babysitter, a musical comedy is running through my head. It's a show about sisters, a vibrant soundtrack that I just can't place. I try to push it aside and tell the babysitter I want her to make "pasta" for dinner, but as I say the words, I know that I intended to say "noodles." I interpret the aphasia as a sign of having had a small lunch.

Another time, I'm preparing dinner when my attention is seized by the presence of an older woman who is caring for a little boy. (To be clear, I'm alone in the house.) I can't discern her words but I feel the entire scene near me, as if it's on television in the other room, as if I've watched the episode so many times that I don't need to hear the dialog at all. I continue setting the table, cut up a pineapple, and chug a glass of water. Eventually, I'm restored to normal.

Are these symptoms? I've learned to move through life believing that the first year after brain surgery is inherently strange. Other than the fact that these episodes all have an auditory component, there are no other patterns that tie them together and I barely register that they're related. What would I tell a doctor anyway, that I periodically have song obsessions and, oh, now I might sense old lady ghosts?

On the day of my one-year checkup, we drive to UCSF and take the elevator to the brain tumor floor, where Jennifer Viner is waiting. She asks generally about headaches and sleep, then conducts the classic neuro tests. I walk in a straight line. I smile and frown. I cite the year and (sadly) the president. When she's finished with my exam, I tell her about the random auditory moments.

"Oh," she says nonchalantly, typing. "It sounds like you're having seizures."

Seizures? Is she serious? I've never considered the possibility of a second diagnosis because the tumor was benign! This shit was over!

Per usual, Jennifer Viner is calm and beautiful and reassuring. She writes me a referral and so, two weeks later, we are back in the same UCSF building, same eighth floor, to meet the next character in my story. Enter epileptic neurologist Dr. Tina Shih.

———

Progress Notes
Tina T. Shih, MD at 5/8/2017 2:30pm
Subjective:

Jennifer Dary is a 36 y.o. right-handed female referred for evaluation of possible seizure disorder. She was accompanied by her husband to this visit.

On 2-15-2016, Jen presented with increasingly severe postural headaches and word-finding difficulties and was found to have a large left sphenoid wing meningioma. She underwent preoperative angio-embolization, then resection in April 2016 and was doing well. She was discharged immediately postoperatively on Keppra and after several weeks was instructed to discontinue without incident. She remembered not feeling well on Keppra and Decadron with irritability and mood problems but wasn't sure which medication was the reason. This resolved once both medications were discontinued.

Starting in August 2016, she has had three stereotyped events. Typical events begin with a sudden sense of being pulled into an auditory memory, e.g. her brain is behind glass, she hears a song or a clip from a podcast or a musical theater in her head; she feels close to identifying this auditory memory. There is a strong sense of familiarity with this experience. It has happened three times in the past year. Sudden onset. Intense from the beginning, then fades away. When it is happening, it is very distracting. She can't have a detailed complex conversation but never has any impairment of awareness. She talks a little slower and a little more deliberately and has to concentrate to come up with the right words.

She denies any episodes of unresponsiveness, confusion, loss of time, subjective sensory events, unexplained self-injury, or incontinence.

The patient was an excellent historian with normal speech/language including naming of low frequency objects and repetition of complex sentences.

Visual fields were full to confrontation, EOMI without nystagmus, facial expression was symmetric.

There were no involuntary movements or tremors.

There was no pronator drift. Rapid successive movements and fine finger movements were symmetric and normal.

Finger-to-nose and heel-to-shin were intact.

Gait was normal.

Plan:

We had an extensive discussion concerning the differential diagnosis and all her questions were answered to her satisfaction. We reviewed the pros/cons of treatment and management options. We decided to hold off on treating with anticonvulsant medications.

I counseled the patient that she can drive. Additional counseling concerning seizure safety was discussed with the patient and her husband and documented in the after-visit summary.

We discussed family planning/teratogenicity of AEDs.

She knows to contact me if she experiences any more events, especially if the events are more severe or result in impairment of awareness.

Total time: 45 minutes

Counseling time: 23 minutes

According to Dr. Shih, it's possible that a tiny bit of scar tissue is left behind after brain surgery. My tumor was right next to my auditory processing center and the place where I store memories. As a result, every once in a while my brain wigs out, realizing that the giant brain tumor it once knew is gone—and that's when I have an auditory-related seizure.

There's no way to predict it, there's nothing that brings it on, there's no food I could cut out of my diet to stop it. My instructions are that I can only have two drinks of alcohol, I must prioritize good sleep, and I am not to take a bath or go into a hot tub if no one else is home.

I message Dr. Shih that night with some questions, still not believing there isn't an obvious solution to this new problem:

1. Why do some people shake when having seizures?

2. How long do they last? Is it just a second or is it until I can think of the lyric, etc.?

3. Would meditation help relax my mind to avoid seizures?

She writes back the next day:

1. Whether someone shakes with a seizure depends on the area of the brain that is involved in the abnormal electrical activity. If the electrical activity spreads to motor cortex, then the patient may have stiffness or shaking.

2. Seizures can last anywhere from a split second up to several minutes. Sometimes it is hard to know how long a single person's seizure is lasting without recording the seizure on EEG. Frequently, the patient's seizure lasts only 1-2 minutes, but they remain confused or impaired for many minutes afterward and that impairment is due to temporary disability in the cerebral cortex involved in the seizure, but the abnormal electrical activity has already subsided.

3. Mindfulness exercises can help many symptoms, but probably not seizures.

Well, shit. Yoga can't get me out of this one. For a while, I'm good at tracking my seizures in an app and I always mention them to Chris, but then life floods in and I stop documenting. Sometimes I say a quick prayer, but the episodes are so rare, so slight, they fade into the unremarkable. Like having the hiccups, seizures are nothing worth noting.

CHAPTER 23

WE DECIDE TO get Aaron baptized. Noah was baptized when he was only a few months old, but we've missed the infant window for Aaron and now he's too big to wear Steve's old baptism suit. Instead, I buy him a collared shirt and khaki pants from Old Navy. Fancy. We ask Leigh to be his godmother.

In my family, godparents were some combination of your aunts and uncles and I assumed godparents' roles were to step in if your parents died, but after growing up and having kids of my own, I feel differently. Godparents are people who are in your life but clearly not your parents—and in this way, they will be safe people for my kids to go to, always. Even if/when our kids go through periods when they assume that Chris and I are idiots, they'll have responsible, loving grown-ups attached to our family to consult with about life.

On the day of Aaron's baptism, the bishop happens to be visiting All Souls. We are asked to meet with him and the other candidates for baptism in the rector's office before the service. Alongside Aaron will be an elderly man, teenage twins, and a baby. I'm nervous that they're going to call Leigh in and grill her, ask her about her faith in God. Her faith is "maybe," which is Chris's faith, too.

What is my faith? It changes. Some days, when I'm fuzzy about my own relationship with The Bigness, I think: it's okay if none of the God stuff is real, I can make up the difference here. I can act from a place of magic; my belief can make the world beautiful for someone else. But this morning we're in a church and we have to renounce the devil and Aaron's wearing white and here is Bishop Marc, wearing a heavy robe stitched with shiny thread. We head into the sanctuary for the service and, frankly, I just want it to be over.

If he was as tiny as Noah was at his baptism, maybe Aaron would squawk a little at the water, but now he's a big guy. I hold him on my hip and the congregation circles around us to watch. Everyone is smiling. The bishop dips his hand in the water and pours a few drops on Aaron's temple. The first time, Aaron is confused. The second time, he glares. The third time, Aaron screams: "I DON'T WANT THIS WATER!" Everyone busts out laughing, Bishop Marc included. For years afterward, this becomes a hilarious and accurate story about Aaron Dary and the strength of his convictions. Despite the rank of those around him, Toddler Aaron will resist pressure and let you know what he needs.

Today, we are playing Dino Family in the living room, a pretend game with Aaron's beloved dinosaur figurines. Some are large, nearly half his height, others tiny enough to fit in his palm. He knows the long names, the plesiosaur and the Compsognathus, the brachiosaur and of course, his favorite, T. rex. He knows the carnivores from the herbivores, the swimmers from the flyers, but when we play Dino Family they all act very human. This morning, the dinos are at a swimming pool and the four brothers are splashing when Aaron suggests a problem.

"How about if that one is having too much fun?"

"Too much fun?" I say. "That's not a thing! That sounds awesome."

"No," he says. "It's too much. The other brothers want a turn."

My mind goes instantly from worrying that my child has a stifled, repressed ability to feel joy to realizing that this is a lesson on sharing. I make the mommy dinosaur gently tell the baby T. rex to come out of the Frisbee pool, and Aaron is delighted when baby T. rex throws a tantrum. He watches, enthralled, as baby T. rex stomps around the pool, even pushes his mommy!

"Oh boy, he needs a time out," I say. On the way to time out, baby T. rex tells his uncle he's a bad uncle, a slick parenting move on my part because lately Aaron has been using this insult on me and Chris. Aaron's eyebrows raise when he hears this; he takes a big breath in and cannot help a slightly scared grin from spreading across his face.

"Baby T. rex, I know you're frustrated but you must use your words," the mommy dino says. "Take a break and then we can invite you back into the pool when you're calm enough to talk."

Our attention moves back to the other brothers, who have found spots in the Frisbee, and a few minutes later we integrate a calmer T. rex back into the fold. This game is a ruse, a school wherein Aaron is studying human dynamics and measuring what's appropriate as we go. At times, he is a nearly silent participant in this game, as if he's watching a movie or listening to a story.

Here are the ways you might see people act, he learns. *Here's the math behind families; here's how to make people in your life a little more predictable. Here are the instructions you wish you had received when you were born. Now you know.*

⁓

"Do you need anything else from downstairs?"

"I think we're good," I say. "Thank you."

The waitress adjusts a few chairs so they offer a better view of the large screen on the wall. We're in the upstairs room of a restaurant in Brooklyn and today is the first day of So Now You're a Manager, a class I've been dreaming about teaching since founding Plucky four years ago. Attendees will start arriving in a few minutes; some of them paid, many of their tickets were comped, but all of the attendees will arrive and stare at me for two days as I teach them what I know about the human side of management.

This is the first time I'm running my own event so I'm a little jittery, but also I don't want people to like this workshop because they pity me. I haven't yet realized that my big life story is a key part of *why* I'm able to put good work into the world. For now, I'm stuck in the mindset that my big life story might be a *distraction* from my work, a version of imposter syndrome that I've never had before.

They're giving you a pass because you almost died. This workshop is a waste of time, but they'll never tell you.

You know, helpful mental gymnastics like this.

Other than being a joy to teach, SNYAM is a strategic move. Building a manager training program—and community—will get Plucky in front of many companies and different people. With Plucky Institute as my north star, I know that I'll need three things to get there: funding, land, and outreach. Funding and land are feeling extremely vague, so I focus on getting my classes out there as broadly as possible.

When I'm teaching a workshop, I often bring someone up from the audience to do a live coaching session. It only lasts about twenty minutes so we aren't able to go too deeply, but, if everything is aligned, the volunteer has an issue that's ripe for action, a reason he raised his hand in the first place. I bring the volunteer up to the front of the room and we sit casually, facing each other while the room watches. After he has laid out the challenge with his boss,

I pause my volunteer client and turn to face the crowd.

"Do you hear what he's saying?" I ask. "Someone tell me, what's *really* going on underneath the boss conversation?"

Attendees call out suggestions. Trust issues? Resentment about his salary? His manager isn't listening to him? Some of these answers are spot-on and others are guesswork, but the validity doesn't need to be 100 percent. What I'm teaching the room is how to listen beyond someone's words.

If we read the transcripts of what happens during meetings, we would only have a two-dimensional perspective because the energetic complexity of a sales call or job interview is masked far below the language. Successful managers see what's invisible to others and use these observations to resource, plan, and motivate teams. Great managers are the most valuable asset a company can have. The opposite is also true.

Next, I ask the room what they're noticing from my volunteer's body language.

"He's all curled up!" "He looks scared!" "He's tapping his foot nervously!"

These cues speak to my volunteer's state of mind, and the other attendees are right to pay attention to these signs. I confide that I haven't pressed him too deeply because I can tell he isn't ready for giant action yet. Then I turn back to him and ignore the rest of the room to resume our session.

"Okay, so let's say you might eventually decide to leave the manager or the company," I say. "That would be a big move. What tiny action do you feel ready for today?" Relief spreads across his face.

"I want to speak up in our next meeting and share my opinion," he declares. "I want to show that I know what I'm doing."

"Great. You can say yes, no, or counteroffer: Will you use your voice at least once in the next team call?"

He consents and we schedule accountability details to make sure it happens. Then we applaud our volunteer as he finds his seat because it's brave to share in front of his peers, and his story allowed all of us to learn. To finish, I pull the lesson together for the room. I ask what they'll take away to use with their employees, if they can tell what's going to happen to our volunteer's story in six months or a year. Having the right answer, again, is not the goal of this exercise. I'm teaching a room full of managers how each individual employee is giving them signs and the importance of tracking motivation and performance, leadership qualities, and burnout. Like Aaron, they are glued to the story.

Here are the ways you might see people act, I teach. *Here is the math behind teams; here is how to make people in your workplace a little more predictable. Here are the instructions you wish you had received when you were promoted into management. Now you know.*

I shouldn't have started oatmeal at 7:10am. It wasn't finished until 7:40, and then it took a while to cool off and the kids had to wolf it down and then I had to rush them through shoes and teeth-brushing and backpacks and show-and-tell choices and then we didn't get to the car until 8:01, which meant traffic was bad on Gilman and we have to wait for all these cars to go through the stop sign and now, instead of our normal routine, we'll have to drop Noah off first.

This is what's happening in half my brain. Simultaneously, the other half of my brain is seizing.

Cajoling. Chiding. She's singing a song snippet, something you learn when you're a kid. This lady caregiver is joking, loving.

Am I thinking about this seizure? Or is it happening? It's like reliving a childhood memory that isn't mine.

Nauseous. Anxious. Driving. Still, the singing. Colors, as though they're shining through bubbles or thin glass. I am beyond time.

It's too powerful to be a memory, too alive. Brought on by stress? I pull up another car-length toward the stop sign. Damn it.

Haze, now. Some fatigue.

We drop Noah off near the front gate, then I take Aaron to pre-school. By the time I'm hugging him goodbye, the seizure has long since passed. I return home to start a day of coaching.

Later, I try to retain words about seizing, but it's like recounting a dream; as soon as you try to describe it, the experience is destroyed. There's usually the familiar singing and a song that I nearly recognize. I'm always being mildly reprimanded by an Eastern European grandmother but also held in love. I never know what she's saying to me but I *feel* her words. The feelings are what stay with me, long after.

Where is God during seizures? I start to have doubts, limiting how often I pray for help because I don't know how many more times I'll need it. *Don't use your panic up on something trivial,* I think. *Save your calls for the next crisis. Always keep something in the tank.*

As if requests of God are finite.

CHAPTER 24

WHEN MY ALARM goes off at 7am Eastern time, my Pacific-time body groans, and it takes all of my effort to reach for my phone and turn it off. From this forgettable hotel bed, I discover a late-night email from my client's CEO that shoots adrenaline into my heart. He is freaking out, unsure of the value of my work, dubious about letting me fly in and teach his staff for the next two days. I patiently respond and tell him that I'll head into the office early so we can talk before I meet his team. I skip the bus and walk to the office, using the mile to regulate my own nervous system.

Comforting senior leadership is part of my job. Executive teams get nervous when you're teaching their staff, as if I'll hear the dirty secrets and judge them for not doing better. Sometimes I *am* disappointed that they've let their own personal issues trickle onto the teams they lead, but disappointment is not productive. I'm there to find ways for everyone to move forward, to progress.

After reassuring the CEO, I take my place at the podium and look out on twenty-two employees, twelve of whom have their zip-up hoodies tight around their faces. Ah, the engineering managers. I recognize them because they project that they don't have time for my bullshitty, soft-skills workshops.

"Like most things in life," I say, "this is going to be what you make of it." I'm talking to myself as much as to my audience.

As we move into class, they start sharing real feelings and challenges. Yes, it is hard to manage people's happiness. Yes, it is hard to trade the innovative, groundbreaking work for that of an exhausted, well-paid manager. No, it is not easy to lead when you've got a new baby or a sick parent or a thousand other pressures beyond these conference rooms.

I tell them that they still must show up; they still must keep trying. The work of a leader is about doing our best, making hard decisions, and leaning on each other as needed. It takes until afternoon coffee, but I get them all on board, even the engineers, hoodies now down.

After such a stressful teaching experience, I develop a strategy to hold my nerves steady, regardless of how the room welcomes me. What was Dr. McDermott like on the day of my surgery? That was a routine work day for him, but there was still great risk. What do surgeons do when they're about to touch someone's brain? Do they study diagrams? Do they pray? What are the rituals? Then I remember: They wash their hands.

In 1847, a Hungarian physician and scientist named Ignaz Philipp Semmelweis proposed that doctors wash their hands before delivering babies. He had noticed that the doctors' wards had three times the mortality rate compared to those of midwives. Dr. Semmelweis couldn't say *why* the hand-washing helped—this was before germ theory—and all of the other doctors were so offended by his suggestion that he was ridiculed and suffered a nervous breakdown. Rough luck.

Now, in modern times, surgeons must focus on scrubbing nails, hands, and forearms for three to five minutes so that they are totally disinfected before surgery. I imagine that this practice helps more than microbes; it's a meditative moment to focus their minds on the job ahead.

Before my next workshop, I decide to adopt the tradition. The attendees are getting settled in their seats when I take one last trip to the bathroom and scrub in. I wash my hands with extra soap, focusing my mind on the work I'm about to do and making sure I'm not distracted by anything that could affect my presence in the room. I also adapt something I heard in church when I was growing up and keep it in mind while I scrub.

May the words of my mouth and the meditations of my heart be acceptable, I think. *May I do good work.*

With that, I grab the door's handle and throw my paper towel in the trash. I enter the room as a teacher, hands clean, faith in myself firm, ready to go.

~

Sometimes it hits in an unexpected place—like the juice aisle at Target—or at an arbitrary time, like when I'm brushing my teeth.

I am shopping for juice boxes. I am alive.

I am brushing my teeth. I have teeth. I am alive.

That happened, I think. *Life is beautiful. I'm okay.*

But there are also very dark times. Within two years, nearly every adult in my vicinity worries that *they* have a brain tumor. Of course I suspect they're traumatized by me and my story, but what do I know? I never imagined my diagnosis, either.

A few friendships end. One woman confronts me with a version of "you think you're so cool since brain surgery." I don't even know how to respond; her comment ends the friendship for me. Like with any relationship that ends abruptly instead of fading away, I reflect on it for a long time. When does believing in yourself become a threat to others? I can be grateful but not too shiny, special but not too special. I can be quietly faithful and mysterious but

I can't claim to know The Bigness more than anyone else. There are social limitations to sharing my experience.

Years later, another friendship ends for a different reason, almost the opposite. In this case, I've been too resilient and now I can't have a bad day—if I do, this friend will tell me exactly what I need to do to put it right again. I'm Jen Dary, girl with the changed life and I'm a safer story if I solve all my problems, forever and ever, Amen. Over time as I live into my restored health and ordinary life struggles, the circle of people that I can genuinely be myself with shrinks.

Exceptions to this are those wrestling life-threatening diagnoses. Friends of friends are continuously referred to me because their husband has a brain tumor, he has six months to live, would I mind talking to his wife? I call her from our back stoop after dinner, our voices immediately intimate because we don't have time for small talk. We are in Big Talk from the jump. I ask her quiet questions in the dark. What stage is it? How long does he have? How will she get health insurance once he's passed?

With these people, I share my ugliest, most heartbreaking thoughts and, looking back, what I most needed as a patient. I admit that I told Chris it was okay to get married again if I died. Time and again, I'm brought back to the incomparable experience of navigating the greatest ending there is. It's bad. She cries, I cry, I can't fix it. But we can sit here together, sharing our realest thoughts—and, for those moments, neither of us are alone.

———

Tonight, like after particularly long days, I'm getting the kids to bed so Chris can run out to do "an errand." This is our code for "I'm going to the ice cream store and will text you a picture of today's flavors." I'm on the couch when Chris returns with treats: cinnamon for me, pistachio-almond for him.

I need to decide if I'm going to financially invest in a manuscript-writing program. It's been hard to write a spiritual memoir while parenting and building Plucky's business, but the book is still very real. I don't feel pressure; it's almost the opposite, as if God's suggestion has now been fully transferred to me, the project's only advocate. It's on me to make this thing fly.

"So what are you going to do?" Chris asks, scraping the bottom of his cup.

"Ugh. I don't know," I say. "I know I'm supposed to write this book. Or, I *thought* I was. But it's been over two years; isn't it old news at this point? There are so many other tragedies out there . . . why bother anyone with my story?"

Chris knows this is a hedge and he's quiet while I unknot my own feelings. Suddenly I'm swept into a moment of energy.

"But you know what? This manuscript program would give me support and accountability, which I clearly need." I pause. "Honey, if I don't write this book, it will be the only regret I can imagine in my whole life."

"I know you will," he says, patiently. "When you say you're going to do something, you do it."

It's his calm response that convinces me more than anything. Chris, the realist in our duo, is telling me he thinks this is going to happen. If *he* thinks it will happen, it probably will! What a weird, backward way of believing in oneself. He reminds me of recent examples when my stubborn drive pushed me to do new and challenging things at work, like inventing packs of Plucky conversation cards. He's right! When I'm clearheaded and aligned with a risk, very little can stop me. Near-death has bulked up my resilience.

Unfortunately, this clarity is temporary. One month later, I'm again doubting if it's the right time and I need to let the instructor know by Monday. Luckily, we're spending the weekend at an All Souls retreat in Healdsburg, wine country. I'm looking forward to recentering and reflecting.

Bishop's Ranch reminds me of a small college campus: sleeping quarters, lounges, a dining room, volleyball courts, and even Adirondack chairs. I peel away from the group one afternoon, finding a spot on a bench behind the labyrinth. I'm here to get down to business with God.

In front of me is a tall, expansive tree—well, more like two trees. After the first few feet of trunk, two trees emerge, their branches covering a significant area with shade. It hasn't rained in eight months, so the ground beneath is covered with dry leaves; beyond that stretches a field of yellow grass. How does nature do it, continue growing up and out, despite entire seasons of drought? This tree has lasted so long without water, somehow keeping its faith. What a metaphor. I close my eyes, a signal to God that I'm picking up the phone.

"Now," I say, "what's the plan, Stan? I've rebuilt my life but we still have unresolved business. You've given me this book idea—you've also given me a vision of buying land. In what order do these dreams go?"

The trouble with listening for God is that you're never getting efficient answers. I hear wind. I hear people's weekend voices, off in the distance. Then in that thin, dreamy broth beneath my consciousness, I find a message. *You got a seed*, I hear. *You choose what to do with it.*

In this moment, under this double-tree, I completely understand what The Bigness means. Seeds are everywhere. Literal acorns lie underfoot—ideas and visions and dreams, figments at best. Which seeds do I want to pick up? Which do I want to plant and tend to, water and prune? I understand that the book and Plucky Institute are invitations, of a sort, but not required missions. Should I choose to take them and run, I'll find adventure. Should I choose to let them die, it's of no matter. There will always be more.

"All right," I say. "Let's do the book first."

As I knew it would, The Bigness gives a double thumbs-up. I leave the labyrinth with commitment and purpose. The book is now a priority.

———

Noah and I have arrived early to pick Aaron up at preschool. The boys ask if we can stay for a few extra minutes to ride the tricycles in the play yard. Chris is out of town on a work trip and lately I've been traveling nonstop for Plucky, so I lean back on the wooden bench, breathing in the warm Friday afternoon. We've made it through another week.

Suddenly, my eyes stop working and my vision is flooded. The yard around me is a convoluted mix of images, as if two worlds have been superimposed. I quickly close my eyes and open them again to clear it away. Shit. Still there.

This has never happened before.

Is this another brain tumor?

How do I get out of it?

One of the preschool teachers is describing her weekend plans, but I have to stop her.

"Sorry," I say. "Something weird is happening with my eyes."

"Oh," Zoe says. "Okay?"

"I'm having trouble seeing," I try to explain. "I had an operation for a brain tumor a couple years ago so I need to figure out what's going on."

God, how awkward it is to insert such heavy personal information into someone else's sunny afternoon.

"Oh!" she says.

I realize that I can see clearly if I keep one eye closed, as if a wire has been disconnected in my head. Later I'll find out that this was a glitch in my binocular vision: Normally our brains meld two slightly different views and connect them to see a singular image, but mine isn't working. In the moment, it's terrifying. I need to drive the kids home, prepare dinner, wheel the trash cans out, and tuck the boys into bed, but how will I leave the preschool yard if I literally can't see? I make a plan.

First, I ask Zoe if she can get me a glass of water. This is partly because having a glass of water never hurts anything and partly because I need to get rid of her so I can problem-solve the situation, alone.

Next, I keep one eye closed as I make my way to the bathroom. "Stay here and play," I tell the kids. "I'll be right back."

Once in the bathroom, I reopen my second eye. Vision is still messed up. I wash my hands with cold water, splashing my face to wake up my senses. I keep one eye closed and make my way back to the bench, where Zoe has returned with water. I open both eyes to check it again: nope. Still awful.

Every time it's still bad, my mind goes quickly to panicked places in which—*fuck!*—this is now a long-term problem. I keep my left eye closed, drink the whole glass of water, inhale deeply, massage my eyelids. I listen to the sound of my boys' voices as they race Strider bikes around the yard. Eventually I open my eyes and—miraculously—my vision has been restored. I blink a few times, daring it to be a fluke, but I seem to be back to a very cautious normal. With no time to lose, the boys are buckled into their car seats and we're off toward home, where I log the episode in my app and go to bed early.

I can imagine how it must sound to read this. *Her eyes stopped working but she was too busy to see a doctor?* What can I say? My kids needed me. No one covered my sick days at Plucky because I *was* Plucky. I was finally making progress on the book and I didn't want a new problem. I assumed that God still had my back.

CHAPTER 25

MY CLIENT KEEPS cutting herself off, as if she holds a stopwatch designed to beep every ten sentences. She gets rolling, sharing her fears, her anxieties, the troubled state of her industry, and just as the conversation picks up fervor and pitch, she lets it go.

"But you know," she says, "first-world problems."

I watch her pick up the pace, describing a company outing where she found out that she's being paid half of what the men around her earn. Though I maintain neutrality, I'm furious for her. She gets angry, feisty even, but then lays it down again.

"I don't have anything to complain about," she says. "Other people have it much, much worse."

As a coach this can be infuriating to watch play out. It is, of course, my job to help her walk through this dilemma, but humans can be like feral cats; approach them slowly and carefully or they flinch and dart away. Losing my emotions wouldn't be productive for anyone, so I stay patient. I ask questions.

"Were the others at the party worried about their first-world problems?"

She snorts. "No way. The world is theirs and they never stop pushing for what they want." I note that she's also allowed to push, and we consider what self-advocacy might look like. She decides to take this as homework to practice before we talk again.

After a long day of coaching, my clients' emotions have pooled in me, so I take a walk to let it all go. Women are still paid less than men. Managers are still not listening. Working parents are still overwhelmed and everyone is always too hard on themselves. As I walk, I exhale the lingering energy of everyone I worked with that day, letting it dissipate in the afternoon air. I invite my spiritual crew to take over, to heal what I cannot.

"I did my best," I pray under my breath. "My shift is over. Now you're up."

I pass my baton to the Divine.

⁓

Dear Jennifer Dary,

I would like to share the news that after 27 wonderful years of service, Dr. Michael McDermott will be leaving UCSF to become the new Director of the Neurosurgery Department at the Baptist Health Systems in Miami . . .

"Oh no!" I say. Chris and Aaron look up. I've been opening mail while warming soup on the stove, and now I've interrupted Aaron's story about an argument with a friend at school. I try to focus on their conversation, but my mind is racing. *McDermott's leaving?* I haven't seen Dr. McDermott in person since my six-week checkup, three years ago, but he's been reviewing my film every April, signing a letter that says I'm clear and recommending another MRI in a year. I'm caught off-guard by my panic. People leave jobs; I know this better than anyone. But *McDermott*!

When dinner is ready, I hand the parmesan cheese to Chris.

"I gotta get out of here for a bit. This McDermott thing is throwing me."

The streets are dim and I walk aimlessly, sometimes crying loud enough to echo off the houses. Emotions pour out of me, embarrassing, loud, disruptive. *Why am I so sad?* For a few blocks I don't understand, I'm just rattled. And then I start talking to myself, pulling it apart.

"I'm sad because he's leaving and because I like him and because I felt safer with him across the bay," I say. "I'm sad because one day Dr. Mike from LA will leave, and Darflinger, too. And Jennifer Viner already has. And it feels like how it will be when my college professors retire, like the campus that was so special to me is not as special if the same people aren't there anymore."

Now I'm crying about my fifteen-year reunion and how amazing it was to be on campus again last year with my Muhlenberg friends, how maybe the places that are special to me are only special because of the people there.

This makes me feel sad because I realize: If I live long enough, the doctors who cared for me, my professors, all of the big sister and big brother tech industry friends I respect, all of them—all!—will be dead.

And *then* I remember that one day my parents will die, my siblings, my friends, my in-laws—*Chris!*—could all die before me. In fact, my father-in-law, Kim, has just been diagnosed with stage IV pancreatic cancer. I take a knee to the sidewalk for a minute. Sobs! Giant, heaving sobs!

I imagine that one day I may be in a nursing home, alone, with no one who knows me and no one left to visit, just left alone to die, with no special people and no special places anymore. *How am I not volunteering at nursing homes every day?!*

I've turned a street corner and from this spot I can see that the stars are out—Orion and others—and I remember how badly Chris broke down after finding my "in case I don't come back" note to the boys. The idea of being among the stars right now on a cool night, instead of in this flawed and scarred human body, that earlier today earned two crowns on molars . . . somehow the distant stars seem more welcoming than this.

And what if Trump gets reelected? And what if civil unrest grows? And what about the homeless? What about all the mean people, the broken ones, the ones who don't care to make a soft landing for others? I will have to see and experience them every day until I die. I'm humbled, imagining every difficult event I'll have to survive before I pass into the vast peace of death.

I spot a small cardboard box at the end of a driveway; inside are a few books and dishes and a pair of men's shoes. I wonder why the shoes are there, if the man died or if he's too old to wear them anymore, and I cry again at this idea, that he's graduated to slippers for good.

Closer to home now, I notice someone's porch light flickering and I assume a kid is playing with the switch, but when I get closer I see that it's actually broken, flashing so rapidly that it looks wild and upset. I acknowledge this out loud: "I see you." Because I do. Because broken and wild and upset is exactly how I feel.

———

I can't let him go without one last lemon loaf.

McDrizz:

Well, I've heard the news. Miami is a pretty long commute to bring you a Starbucks lemon loaf every April, but I'm not saying it's impossible. I'm going to be at UCSF next Tuesday to do some writing for a few hours. Remember that book I've been working on? It's got a due date! Looks like you'll be a famous neurosurgeon after all . . .

After a few back-and-forths with his assistant, I take an afternoon off work to head to Parnassus. It's Dr. McDermott's last day in the office. The receptionist is apologetic.

"It's very busy," she says. "He's still seeing patients and also so many staff members are coming by; we're having a surprise party for him in the lounge. Plus, sometimes it's hard for him to see former patients . . . he's known people for so long. I think it's making him upset."

"Yeah, well," I say, "that's because he's the literal best."

Knowing that Dr. McDermott might lose it helps me ground my own emotions. If I get to see him, I'm going to go in with a high-five-McDrizz vibe; I will not repeat my nighttime weeping walk. I give the nurse my name and open my laptop while waiting for a possible two-minute gap between his final appointments.

Around me, patients and their caregivers stare out the wall of windows: Mount Tam, the Bay Bridge, a cathedral, Golden Gate Park, and the Pacific Ocean. What must it have been like to see this view every day for twenty-five years? Through presidents and national crises, better and more advanced scientific technologies, tragedy upon tragedy for hundreds of patients. Some who lived, like me; some who didn't. I'm inspired by the impact one human being can make.

I peer at the San Francisco houses below me and consider this city. Here at UCSF Parnassus, I'm far from Market Street, where many of the tech companies live. Before San Francisco became part of Silicon Valley, it was known for other things. Before all of us in this waiting room earned rainbow scars across our heads, we were known for other things, too.

—

"Jennifer?"

The assistant walks me behind the desk where Dr. McDermott looks good, happy, maybe a little overwhelmed.

"You! You were the one with the *big* tumor!" he says. Ah, the ways we are recognized in this weird life. I high-five him and hand him a bag with a lemon loaf and two chapters of this book.

"It's happening," I say. "I'm writing a book about all of this!"

He tells me that he has another patient who went through medical school, became a doctor himself, and now they're making a movie about him, to be released later this fall. The movie stars Brad Pitt.

"What the hell," I say. "I guess that means I'll need someone even hotter to play my husband when we start filming."

McDermott laughs and then, like that, he's off to his next appointment. I feel closure. I'm hoping to come back a few more times to work on the ending of the book, maybe even to visit Dr. Mike from LA. I'll need a specialist's help translating the scientific words about brain surgery and, weirdly enough, I actually like being here. Hospitals—especially UCSF—are places where *everything matters,* where patients are constantly reminded of the limits of their earthly bodies, where angel reps hang around with clipboards, dispensing coincidences and deathbed visions, as required.

On my way out, I stop by the meditation room, a rare place of stillness in these active buildings. Chairs are arranged in a half circle, all facing the image of a large, calming lotus flower. Bibles, prayer cards, holy books, and a yoga mat are in the sliding storage cabinet near the door. On the counter is a worn guest book where you can ask for prayers.

I love the intention of this room, the way The Bigness is embraced so fully, illustrating that there are many, many channels available when it comes to connecting with God. Maybe you are hopeful; maybe you are hopeless. The meditation room says to pick the framing that feels right to you, the one that brings you the most comfort. Miracles through devastation; all are welcome in this room.

CHAPTER 26

I'M FLYING BACK from teaching Plucky's latest manager training. High on the energizing trip, I spend the flight home outlining big plans for my book and for Plucky. The kids are slightly older now, Noah in kindergarten and Aaron turning four, and I'm convinced that we're glimpsing the season that friends with older children have assured me will come, a time when traveling for work isn't a near-impossible ask of your spouse. We've moved into a three-bedroom house. I have a real office. Maybe I can finally dream bigger? Maybe I've finally got the timing right.

At 30,000 feet up in the air, I feel closer to The Bigness and my spiritual committee than I have in a while. I fill my notebook with plans for cities, scaling myself as a trainer, even scaling myself as a coach. I'm going to increase ticket prices, hire other coaches, really build this rocket ship. I craft an ideal writing calendar, blocking out uninterrupted time to write. After all, this is the year of the book. *Book! Plucky Institute!* I think, *I am coming!*

But upon landing, a bundle of texts arrive from Chris, the kind you send under duress when you're aching for the other parent to return quickly. Things at home are not good. Aaron hasn't been sleeping and his tantrums are getting worse, sometimes turning violent. Handling drop-offs and pickups alone has caused a significant amount of work stress for Chris.

I take my bag down from the overhead compartment and sling it wearily over my shoulder as we deplane. Every aspiration recorded during the flight is suddenly a joke.

In the cab ride back to Berkeley, I'm nauseous, also angry. Every moment that I'm needed by a child, every missed homework assignment or unpaid bill, is another nail in the cage-like box I feel I'm in. For Plucky to fly, for this book to happen, certain aspects of my family life must be functional without me. I need time and space away from mothering for my own growth. I thought we were nearly there. Clearly, we are not.

⌣

"Tell me about his first year," says the child psychologist. "Did Aaron have a relatively normal first year of life?"

Chris and I look at each other. We chuckle, the way you prepare a listener for a magnitude for which she is not ready.

"The first eight months were normal," I say. "And then when he was nine months old, I was diagnosed with a brain tumor."

"Oh." Ruth exhales deeply.

I look around for something wooden; the arm of the chair looks good. I do my speech.

"I'm okay now, though," I say. "I had brain surgery and they got it all and it was benign." I knock on the chair's arm for effect.

Ruth's pen is moving quickly. I tell her about the symptoms, the time away from Aaron, the hasty weaning, the family who visited. She asks more questions, gently wondering if my medical history had long-tail effects on others.

A few weeks later, Ruth walks us through her report. She has observed Aaron at school and at home.

"I observe Aaron to be very smart and curious, a child who has busy eyes and a busy brain. He is so alive and engaged with life!" She also notes that he is a high-intensity, high-sensitivity, low-adaptability child. Ruth wonders if some of these temperament characteristics are causing Aaron's sleep issues.

This is ultimately why we're here. Our boy has stopped sleeping. Or, rather, he's lost all rhythm to his sleep. He goes down all right, but then he's awake at 1am, up sometimes for two or three hours. He lies there, eyes wide open, kicking or clearing his throat, refusing to go back to sleep and preventing one of us from leaving the room. We are exhausted—and so is he.

"He just seems angry to be here on the planet," Chris says. "Like he's eternally frustrated with the limitations of being four years old."

Nearly forty minutes into her feedback, Ruth brings up the tumor.

"Aaron was a baby, so he doesn't have memories of it," she says. "But babies read our energy really well and are influenced by it. No doubt, you had many loving people caring for Aaron during that time. But they all were very scared. I think he could be remembering their anxiety without understanding where all that fear came from."

She has other suggestions, all helpful, about handling separation when we drop off at preschool and ways to relax him at night before bed. She encourages us to tell him about times that we're frustrated by our own limitations, like when we're struggling at work or doing something for the first time. But there is, she says, no single answer.

"This may be a difficult period as he grows through this," she says.

A difficult period? Something inside me collapses.

When we get home, I quit everything: church, the PTA, social events, and anything outside the bare minimum for Plucky. Chris and I ground ourselves in routine. We borrow children's library books about processing feelings, how to use your words to express anger, and time outs. We order groceries on Instacart. I turn inward and stop responding to texts. I swallow my plans for Plucky and hide my notebook of grand ideas, even starting a fresh one to record singular to-dos. I keep my dreams minuscule in the crushing way that life sometimes requires us to do.

⁓

Mother's Day 2019, journal entry:
The last few weeks and months have been really difficult. Does it get better than this? Will our home be calm again? Will the burned-out-parenting-firefighter-response let us breathe easier one day? Good God, I fucking hope so.
They never tell you how impossible this is. They never tell you how you will reach cul-de-sacs that you cannot see your way out of. Are we doing the right thing? Is Aaron okay? When do we discipline? When do we let go?
Dear God, please help me to see each moment as an opportunity for new and different. I need some hope.

⁓

After a long week of coaching and parenting, I take the boys to church.

"Let us confess our sins against God."

The congregation moves into action. Depending on preference, some fold the kneelers down in the pews, others remain standing and bow their heads. I never kneel; I didn't grow up kneeling, it strikes me as much too Catholic and I'm never sure how to do it.

I'm also feeling very angry this morning, so my bow is closer to a subversive chin tuck. Noah is antsy next to me in the pew. Aaron looks through a Pokémon book, a stark difference from last night when we fought over bedtime and he told us he wished we were dead.

The assisting minister continues:

"God of all mercy . . ." and then the congregation joins in.

we confess that we have sinned against you

opposing your will in our lives.

One line into confession, I nearly leave the church in protest. I do not have space to hear about my sins this morning.

We have denied your goodness in each other,

in ourselves, and in the world you have created.

Really? I just spent a thankless week coaching, parenting, recycling plastic, donating stuff to Goodwill, and emotionally supporting friends and family from afar.

We repent of the evil that enslaves us,

How can I repent of something that is so much more powerful than I am?

the evil we have done,

Damn it. I have done a lot of things this week. Evil is not one.

and the evil done on our behalf.

Fair enough. Trump is locking children in cages—though I didn't vote for him, so I'm not sure why I have to repent here.

Forgive, restore, and strengthen us through our Savior Jesus Christ,

By this point, I am livid. I don't want to hear about my Savior Jesus Christ. The only interaction I've had with that guy this week is in this church service. Where was he when Aaron was sleepless in the night? And during my family's recent reunion at the Jersey Shore, when it erupted in tension, old baggage, and hurt feelings yet again? Forgive *me*, Savior Jesus Christ? How about we try to forgive *you*?

that we may abide in your love and serve only your will. Amen.

Lately, my entire life is serving someone else's will. Eff off.

After the service ends, I follow the kids to the church playground. Friends see me from afar and carefully ask how I'm doing; they sense I haven't been my usual self. I move coldly through these interactions.

"Fine, good. Thanks." I say all of these, when clearly I mean none.

My friend Nikki, a seminarian, finds me on a bench. I express to her my beef with Jesus.

"I honestly can't say confession right now," I say. "I cannot even utter the words. It feels insulting, so hurtful to where I'm at."

She looks at me, confused.

"I wish confession could be reduced to four words: I tried my best."

Now I'm crying to a future priest on a bench at the church playground, feeling completely vulnerable. Nikki is patient and sweet, but I'm embarrassed and unsure of what I'm even asking, so I sniff a few times, give her a hug, and round up the kids to go home.

As I drive, I wonder: What if it *had* been stress back in 2016? Who would I have become without the tumor? What's the Venn diagram of me, before and after? Wife of Chris. Small business owner. Mother to two sons. New Yorker who moved to California. Brain Tumor Survivor subsumes everything that came before it; it's the only identity that anyone hears. Hell, it's the only one that I hear.

More often than you'd think, I am sick of polishing my trauma, bitter toward the gritty truth that I survived . . . and that maybe this magical survival was a fluke.

CHAPTER 27

SHORTLY INTO THE 2020 New Year, I finally admit that the seizures are becoming a thing and something's up with my eyes. At times, my vision is blurry and my eyes tear up, particularly the left. Not good. I vacillate between guessing that I need glasses and worrying that I've been growing another brain tumor. The next annual MRI is still a few months away, so my neurosurgeon suggests visiting an ophthalmologist. I arrive early for my eye appointment, where an innocent technician declares my early victory.

"Twenty-twenty vision!" she says. "How about that?"

I explain that my situation is a little more complicated than reading glasses, and by the time Dr. Lee arrives in the exam room, I'm convinced that this visit will be like so many others: a waste of precious time. But after I walk him through my medical history, Dr. Lee leans back in his chair.

"Well, when I saw the note that you were feeling pressure in your eyes, I thought you probably had allergies," he says in an interested voice. "But maybe not."

Finally, a challenge for the learned doctor! He leans closer and looks squarely at my face.

"They did a really good job putting things back together, but one eye is a little lower than the other."

Dr. Lee explains that my brain doesn't only have to use binocular vision to mesh together two different images; it also has to bring the discrepancy in heights together. *Damn*, I think, *my poor brain has been doing so much extra work.*

"I think you're doing pretty good neurologically if you're writing a memoir about it all," he continues.

Another reminder of the gift of borrowed time. I feel sick remembering that parenting my kids and running Plucky are major prizes. Field trip permission slips, cat hairballs, infinitely emptying the dishwasher, some new weird sickness called coronavirus. *Why am I letting life's day-to-day stress me out?* Self-judgement abounds.

The nurse puts yellow numbing drops in my eyes and when I wipe them with a Kleenex, it looks like I'm crying out saffron. Dr. Lee pushes his viewing machine close enough to touch my eyeball, to which I flinch.

"Mind over matter," he says. "You're fine, just look here at this white dot."

I get calm and focused, which lets him touch my eyeball's surface. He takes measurements in both eyes.

"Well, you're not making this up. This left eye has twice as much moisture as the right one, which is already more than normal."

"What are you saying?" I ask. "What does that mean?"

"Your eyes are inflamed. I'm prescribing anti-inflammatory drops."

"Like Advil for my eyes?"

Dr. Lee smiles. "Better than Advil. Prednisone." I recognize this name. A steroid. Ugh.

"We'll do a nerve scan today and then you'll come back for a vision field test in a couple weeks. I want us to have a baseline. Frankly, it might have happened much sooner after surgery, but here we are."

Before bed, I shake the tiny bottle and look up. I hit the right eye on the first shot, but the left one takes a couple tries. Only after I succeed do I look back toward the mirror, where a few rogue drops spill down my left cheek. Looks like I'm crying milk.

———

Aaron wanders into my office.

"Noah said something mean to me!" he says, his tears big and sad. I turn away from my computer, where I'm trying to write an email before I take the boys to school. As I walk him back to his cereal in the kitchen, the story comes out.

"Aaron said he can do *anything*," Noah says. "And I told him, 'No you can't. You can't cook.'"

Aaron cries again. "See? That's mean! I *can* do anything!"

It is a tale of older siblings vs. younger siblings, but it's also one of dreams vs. logic.

"Noah, I hear that you're saying logically there are things Aaron can't do right now, but I want you to think about how that makes him feel. He's four years old; it's exciting for him to say he can do anything."

I turn toward Aaron. "Aaron, I know that you can do anything. You're going to do amazing things because you're an amazing kid! You both are."

The discussion descends into pooping and our morning rolls on, but after we drop Aaron off, I bring it up again with Noah.

"Buddy, you know what's something funny about people? If you tell someone that they can't do something when they're young, they believe it for a really long time. Like, if I told you, 'Geez, you're bad at dancing,' and I told you that regularly, it would be nearly impossible for you to drop that belief when you're older."

Noah is thoughtful in the backseat.

"Did anyone tell me bad things when I was little?"

"Not on purpose, no. But maybe me or Dad told you to be careful about something that was scary when you were younger and you'll have a hard time forgetting it. Of course, there are some things that will always be dangerous, like touching a stove or crossing a street without looking. But as you get bigger, you'll be able to do more, too. It's important not to keep these warnings so close that they become beliefs."

We talk about telling girls they're bad at math or first graders that they can't skateboard. Those would be unfair beliefs that would affect large groups of people.

"I coach grown-ups every day who are trying to undo their old beliefs," I say. "I want you and Aaron to start your lives with the most confidence possible. Because I'm not kidding when I say you could do anything in your life, even become a really good president."

Given the moron currently in the White House, I think, *Noah—at seven years old—could do better.*

On my walk back to the car, I mine my own limiting beliefs. Passing parents and grandparents outside the school, I imagine all the limitations that are still influencing their lives today.

So many people, I think as I pull the car onto the street. *So many people trusting so many voices besides their own.*

⁓

Summer 2020. Chris brings in the last of the bags from Target and immediately goes to the bathroom to wash his hands. I start the routine for putting groceries away:

First, wipe down the item with Clorox wipes.

Second, put the item on a dish towel to dry off.

Last, put the items away in the cabinets and fridge.

Clorox wipes are running low at every store, so I reuse each cloth for multiple items. The stores are out of toilet paper, hand sanitizer, milk, bread, and more. I move my sourdough starter aside to make room for the eggs. I barely recognize the brands these days because you buy whatever they have. These are the times of early coronavirus.

The kids have been out of school for two months. What at first felt like a freewheeling couple of weeks as fun substitute-teacher-parents is now the burden of reality. Chris and I maneuver our schedules so that I coach my East Coast clients early before he starts work, then I tack on a few more hours in the late afternoon while the kids watch a movie. Every single moment of the day is a responsibility.

But besides the schedule, it's also terrifying. Can you get Covid from surfaces? What if you pass by a person who just coughed? There are so many questions and, at this point, very few answers. All we know is *other people are bad.* We pine for takeout to avoid cooking another freaking dinner, but there's no way we'd eat food prepared by someone else. Playgrounds are dangerous, school is closed, we are adjusting to the first incarnation of distance learning, and it's awful. To our credit, we know how to do emergencies. Like zombies, we simply stay the course and swallow all panic.

Meanwhile, in Wisconsin, Kim is nearing the end of pancreatic cancer. Despite potential clinical trials, my father-in-law's body is not the right match for the remaining options. Hospice starts coming to their house. We text photos to Beth: the boys climbing a tree, digging holes at the beach, being silly with our new kitten.

During Kim's final few days, I send Beth an audio recording of the kids chatting over lunch and 20 minutes of happy home background noises. I hope she can play it for Kim as he rests, a crappy replacement because we can't be together.

We move into July holding him in our minds, on edge, a nervousness that envelops anticipation. *Someone is leaving soon, maybe today.* We spend the hours in mental flight, circling, waiting for this life transition to land. As with birth, the timeline of death is out of human control. Kim's leaving cannot be postponed.

———

"Did they show a gravestone?"

"Not that I could see, just a picture on a stand."

We're bounce-passing a tired old tennis ball back and forth while the boys ride bikes around the basketball courts. Chris is still wearing a button-down shirt, the one he changed into for the service this morning. I imagine it's hard to know what to wear to your dad's funeral when it's being conducted on FaceTime.

The shadows are long across the blacktop, our mood quiet and final, the way summer Friday evenings during this pandemic tend to be. The week is done. A father's life is done. Now there's just the soft pinging of a tennis ball, passed back and forth to cushion the weight of such a day.

Soon after Kim's death, I drive the boys to a cemetery up the hill near El Cerrito. I feel like a trespasser as I pull into the small parking lot, but no one knows that our recent loss is halfway across the country. We walk along paths and across lawns and around graves and I tell the boys about cremation, burials, and caskets. I show them how to spot clues like mason symbols or military icons. We talk about why a two-year-old would die in 1924, why some headstones are tiny and why others are small buildings. We imagine what Grandpa's grave might look like in Wisconsin and what kinds of flowers we might bring once the pandemic is over.

The breeze blows our words around the hills and this outing is as important as almost any church service we've attended. On this summer afternoon, when I might have otherwise been working, it's just me and the boys, exploring what happens when we leave our bodies. One day, Bigness-willing, they will visit my grave. I beg The Bigness for our deaths to go in that order.

Keep them safe, I pray. May they live long, long lives that surpass us. *Amen. Amen. Amen. Amen.*

———

Where is God during a pandemic? During the death of a father? Despite the chaotic landscape, I'm hoping that magic still exists, but church has been canceled and lately I'm struggling with where to find The Bigness. For months, I string my faith along with small prayers and tarot cards. It's barely enough to get through these parched days, and I long for a huge gulp, a giant sign of proof.

Bigness, reassure me. Has this all been for nothing?

Things are about to get worse.

CHAPTER 28

*RED FLAG WARNING FOR THE EAST BAY HILLS; NO
PSPS PLANNED FOR BERKELEY*
*The National Weather Service has issued a Red Flag Warn-
ing for the East Bay Hills for Wednesday at 10:00pm through
Friday at 8:00am. Fires that start during Red Flag Warnings
can spread quickly.*
*Leave your phone turned on so you can be alerted, even if you
are sleeping.*
Put your go-bag by the front door.
*Review your household's evacuation routes. Make sure to plan
at least two routes away from your neighborhood. During an
evacuation you may not be able to drive, so consider using the
network of Berkeley Path Wanderers in your evacuation plans.*
*Park off-street. Back your car into your driveway or garage,
leaving streets clear for emergency vehicles.*
Reply with YES to confirm receipt.

We reply YES to confirm receipt of every alert, sometimes three
in a day. Public Safety Power Shutoffs, rolling blackouts, smoke
from regional fires, air quality alerts, prepare for high winds and fire
danger. We ask neighbors for advice about go-bags and evacuation

routes, but even our native Californian friends are lost. They didn't grow up with these fires, either.

The temperature outside climbs to the 90s, but we can't open the windows to catch a breeze because the smoke is so thick. Here in temperate Berkeley, we don't have air-conditioning and it's *hot*. After a particularly bad week of awful air we consider driving south for a night, but by the time we're ready to leave, the smoke has reached our destination, too. It's not worth driving five hours to quarantine with the same four people in a tiny hotel room, so we cancel.

Then, it's the day of no sun.

At 9am on September 9, 2020, it looks like it could be 9pm. Smoke blowing in from multiple fires has converged, the sun is hidden, and the streets are ghostly gray. I step onto the front steps wearing a scratchy white N95 mask. Not one bird noise, not even a slight wind. The stillness is so solid that it's like being on a stage, on a set, where a show has ended and everything has been put away. Even the photos I'm taking to send to my mom and Steve can't capture the reality because my iPhone keeps adjusting the lighting, and it's a losing battle to show how scary things really are.

Something deep within me says: *enough*.

I haven't talked about my desire to leave California with almost anyone because I don't want family members back east to get their hopes up, and I don't want friends and family out west to get offended, but deep in my bones, I've known that California is not where we're supposed to be.

I'm going to take a shower, I text to Mom and Steve. *More soon*.

The shower is the only place I'm alone these days. Instead of smoke, I smell Ocean Breeze body wash. I turn the hot water up so it's burning the top of my head, my shoulders, my back. For a moment, I can convince myself that I'm living another day in another time.

"Listen up, Bigness," I whisper. "This is serious. I'm ready to leave but I don't know where we should go next. I really, really need a sign. Preferably a zip code."

Of course, I assume my prayer will go nowhere. Why would today be different?

I make my way to the bedroom to get dressed and, on the way, grab my phone from the kitchen table. Steve has sent three texts.

The first says, *You know, we have good air in Virginia . . .*

The second is a link to a house for sale near him in Alexandria.

The third says, *Oops, how did this get here? ;)*

I stare at the ceiling in disbelief. *Virginia?*

Never, *never,* have I been interested in moving to the DC area. We don't work in government and I don't want to live anywhere near Trump. But I asked The Bigness for a location and I got one.

"Ha!" I respond lightly to Steve, because he has no idea the impact of his joke, but inside my mind is racing.

Is Plucky a Virginia company? Are my kids Virginians? Is Virginia still considered The South?

This is a twist I never expected.

After an anxious day, night comes and the darkness is not out of place. I meet Chris on the couch.

"Hear me out," I say. "I have to show you a text from Steve."

The idea of leaving expands in the room, dangerous in its appeal. It's illuminating to see what kinds of rentals we could afford outside the Bay Area. More space, a yard, clear skies, all for less money than we're paying in Berkeley. For the first time since the pandemic started, we hold a modicum of control. *We could pull this off!* The air in the room shivers.

"I'm in," Chris says immediately. "Let's get out of this stank hole."

Logistics abound. Can Chris work remotely for Reddit? Can the kids stay in Berkeley distance learning for the foreseeable? Are we moving to Alexandria? Arlington? DC? Some other unknown town?

The move propels us upward, an invitation to return to the East. We're motivated by the prospect of reconnecting with family, friends, to live within driving distance of New York! Green grass and a yard and hot summers and snowstorms—woo! If I can accept the idea of moving to Northern Virginia, this sounds so damn good.

We make a spreadsheet and think through all angles: the cost of the move, a bigger rental home, the impact on our careers by leaving the Bay Area. These questions are mostly due diligence, but we know we have to ask; we won't leave spontaneously and upend our kids' futures without intention. We play it out, all kinds of scenarios, but three weeks later, moving is officially the plan.

One friend asks "Are you moving *away* from something or *toward* something?" and with such a slippery question, I'm not sure which is correct. I think the answer is: both.

⁓

The moving POD has left. Our car is on a transporter, already nearly across the country, and Steve will pick it up for us tomorrow. We are spending our last California afternoon at Kate's, celebrating her daughter's fourth birthday a month early. Chris and I leave the boys with Kate for an hour while we shop for airplane snacks. Flying cross-country in a pandemic will mean masks the whole way, lots of hand washing, only eating the food we bring with us onto the plane. We get one last coffee at Peet's.

"How are you feeling?"

"Good," Chris says. "Ready to go. You?"

I am not sad. I'm sure that one day I will miss things about our life here (people, specifically), but we said a weird version of goodbye eight months earlier in March when everything closed down.

It's easier to leave because this grief is not new. It's also easier to leave because we have something exciting awaiting us on the other side, our *next*.

"Same," I say. "I'm ready, too."

The next morning: a thousand little moments, like levels in a video game. Return rental car at the airport. NEXT LEVEL. Get through metal detectors with the cat. NEXT LEVEL. Set the kids up with fully charged tablets and headphones. NEXT LEVEL.

It's a long flight to DC, but I can't read or watch TV, hyper-aware of our masks, proactive about bathroom breaks, the kindest version of myself because we don't need drama. Yes, have another lollipop, yes, another juice is fine, another episode of that show? Sure! I watch the plane icon move east across the map of America toward a soon-to-be President Biden. Goodbye California, Colorado, Midwestern states. Hello Pennsylvania, hello the *familiar*. Soon enough, we're getting ready to land and I can't believe we made it, the cat and the kids and everything, all the levels we checked off today. Outside my window is the Washington Monument, the simple visual enough to bring tears to my eyes. *Hello, new friend.*

But I don't have time to get too sentimental; we still have a few levels to go! Rental car, NEXT LEVEL. Find keys from Steve for the new house, NEXT LEVEL. Pull into our driveway—our driveway!—and absorb our large backyard and front stoop, unlock our front door. FINAL LEVEL ACHIEVED.

From somewhere far away (but not so far, never so far), my angel rep nods. We have been guided. I've felt her and The Bigness and their team with us the whole way.

CHAPTER 29

NEARLY A YEAR after our move to Arlington, I prioritize finding a local neurologist. Referred by my primary care doctor, I wait several months to meet with Dr. Carroll. My health hasn't changed; seizures may be a little more frequent, but having partial focal seizures is like being double-jointed. A creepy party trick, nothing more.

Arriving at his office, I'm weirdly excited to meet the Virginia version of Dr. McDermott, who will surely address my medical history with reverence and smarts.

"Why am I seeing you?" Dr. Carroll says. A brisk start, but I roll with it.

"Are you a neurologist?"

"Yes, but why aren't you seeing a neurosurgeon?"

Now I'm confused. *Neurosurgeons* sound like doctors you see when you need brain surgery. *Neurologists* sound like doctors who take care of your brain when it plans to stay safely inside its skull. Maybe this guy doesn't realize I've already had brain surgery?

"I had a craniotomy in 2016 for a meningioma," I explain patiently. "So that's all taken care of! But I'm here today because we just moved from California last fall and I need to find a local doctor."

Without a word, Dr. Carroll sits down at his computer and starts typing.

"I see that. I see it was resected at UCSF. You wrote that you're having seizures, but you didn't write what medication you're on."

"Oh, I'm not on seizure medication," I say. "I saw a neurologist who specializes in epilepsy in 2017, but she thought they were mild and we didn't need to medicate."

"You're telling me you've had seizures for four years and you're not on seizure medication? You're telling me you have seizures and you're still driving?"

This guy is starting to piss me off.

"That's what I'm telling you."

"No one ever did an EEG on you?"

"No."

"You're telling me that no one ever glued electrodes to your head and measured your brain activity?"

I know what a fucking EEG is. I think I would remember that happening.

"No one ever did that," I say. In the tense silence, my inner advocate rises up.

"I'm going to be honest," I say. "I'm feeling really defensive right now. I'm simply showing up to establish care and somehow I feel like I've given all the wrong answers. We may not be the best match."

I put my hand on the chair to get up, unsure if this conflict is going to escalate.

"Do you lose control of your bladder? Do you lose consciousness?"

This fool just keeps going down the list of seizure side effects, immune to my suggestion that he is acting aggressively and that I—the patient!—am not happy about it.

I don't know why I stayed. Maybe it was because we were only three minutes into an appointment for which I'd waited three months. Maybe it was because *his* alarm was causing *me* alarm. Maybe it was because my seizures were happening more lately and I was worried that a doctor knew my body better than I did, a scary echo of 2016.

"No," I say. "No to both of those."

Dr. Carroll rolls on with basic questions about my side effects. He has me stand up and do the classic neuro tests. Put your arms out like you're holding a pizza box. Push on my fingers. Walk in a straight line. Balance on one foot. Eventually he leaves the room to print something out and when he comes back I am standing, arms crossed, staring at his wall of diplomas. I've planned for him to catch me here, doubting him and his pedigree. I am flipping the power in the room.

"Why did you go into neurology?"

He's typing on the computer as he answers. "I like anatomy and complex problems."

No mention of humans. No mention of patients. I don't care what this guy ultimately recommends; the only way forward for me is a second opinion.

He tells me to start anti-seizure medication that night. He gives me samples—samples!—of a medication with serious side effects, including depression and suicidal tendencies. He schedules me for an EEG in his office a month from now and refers me to an epilepsy neurosurgeon. On my way out the door, I throw his referral in his trash. Who accepts referrals from *assholes*?

———

As I call around for second opinions, I come to understand that, this time, I'm not important at all. I write to folks at the Johns Hopkins Meningioma Center. I ask UCSF for a DC-based referral.

Between coaching calls, I spend hours leaving messages and faxing records. I even consider contacting Dr. McDermott, who's still based in Miami. I can't seem to move this forward at all, plus now the kids are back in school, which impacts how fast I can accomplish health chores.

Though I want to cancel Dr. Carroll's EEG, Chris and I agree that it would be a good asset to have in-hand when we find a new doctor. I do not, however, fill the anti-seizure prescription at the pharmacy and I don't start taking Dr. Carroll's samples. Medication feels like a huge decision, and I don't want to make it without another doctor involved.

On the morning of the EEG, I prep my materials to teach manager training later in the day and get the kids off to school. Once in Dr. Carroll's office, a kind nurse named Mary tells me that I won't see the doctor during my appointment. I tell her that's good news, that I think he's a shitty excuse for a doctor, and she attempts to hide a smile.

"Don't think about any of that now," she says. "Today is a new day."

Nurse Mary has me lie back on the table. She stands above my head and tapes electrodes to my scalp. She hangs a bright light a few inches above my face and takes a seat at the desk.

"Okay, I'm all set," she says. "I'm going to get it started, and it should only last about thirty minutes. You good?"

"Yeah, I'm okay," I say. *Bigness, be with me.*

"Close your eyes," she says. "It's going to start now."

The first thing that happens is an intense flashing of lights. They flash to no rhythm, repeat with no pattern, and, despite the fact that my eyes are closed, they're bright. I don't like this. After a few seconds, it ends.

Phew, I think. *That was rough.* The backs of my eyelids are a relief, but soon the flashes start again. This time, the sequence is faster and more intense and the lights are more blinding. Each time it ends, there's a short break and then the lights come on again, rapid, scary, wildly out of pattern. This EEG feels dangerous, the way your stomach drops when you're driving too fast around a curve or going over a really big bump on your bike. I grip the pockets of my jeans and hold on, teetering on the edge of too-stimulated. What gives it a particularly torturous vibe is that, each time, the sequence is longer and brighter and more frantic than the last.

May this be over, I beg. *May this be the last time.* But it isn't, not for a while.

I don't notice any seizures, but apparently the machine does, because Dr. Carroll leaves me a rude voicemail saying that seizure activity was present in my left temporal lobe, the location where the tumor was removed. He tells me to increase the dose of the seizure meds that I never started in the first place. At the end of the message, he tells me that I shouldn't be driving.

Fuck you, I think. Even still, I have a bad feeling about this recommendation.

The next day, I check our mailbox to find that my new Virginia driver's license has arrived, and with it, a letter from the DMV Medical Advisory Board.

Dear Jennifer Dary:

The Department of Motor Vehicles (DMV) is in receipt of information concerning your ability to safely operate a motor vehicle . . .

According to this letter, my driver's license will be suspended at the end of the month unless I provide documentation from a doctor that confirms I'm *not* having seizures. Immediately, I assume that Dr. Carroll reported me, but then I realize: It wasn't him. It was *me.* When I applied for a Virginia license last month, I filled out a medical report. *Have you ever had a seizure, blackout, or loss of consciousness?* Without hesitation, I checked *yes.* For me, the seizures have always been strange little blips, but apparently they're significant to everyone else, including, now, the state of Virginia.

———

Parenting, pandemics, wildfires, politics . . . somehow this crisis is different. Those trials were external, circumstances that I was interacting with, but now, for the second time, I'm the circumstance.

Friends send frozen meals, boxes of cheese, gift cards, and flowers; everyone is holding me carefully during this time. Maybe to the outside world it looks like I have an insatiable ability to reframe and find purpose, but in the lonely night hours, I lie under heavy shadow. There are times I wonder how bad it would be if seizures led to the end, how tiring it is to stay positive, how warm and welcome it might be to put this weight down.

Though I've been calling Georgetown for weeks without a response, I finally get through the next day and the nurse gives me an appointment for later that week.

Thanks, I whisper skyward. *Get me to the right doctor, get me to someone who is not an asshole.*

We're headed to the appointment when doubt swoops in, maybe even fear. What if they put me on meds while we're in the office and I forget who I am or how to be? I tell Chris I need to run back upstairs, grab a pen and document the truest things I know about myself. I write as fast as I can.

In case meds change me, remember that:

I am happy.

I find joy in lots of things, like dogs and cats and bookstores and stationery sections and friends and traveling and learning and libraries and dinner parties.

I get stressed by: family and disappointing others. Feeling too alone.

I like: cheese, sweet breakfasts, chai lattes, coffee with milk, cake, fancy salads, everything bagels with veggie cream cheese.

I don't like: mushrooms, pickles, fish, fake or pompous people.

If I lose myself, I can refind me: in Egner Chapel, at Bishop's Ranch, on Court Street in Brooklyn, walking the loop around my neighborhood in Arlington.

I believe in: God, spirit guides, an afterlife + magic.

I make the best of things.

I am creative.

I love so much.

Me, documented. Just in case.

CHAPTER 30

FROM THE OUTSIDE, Medstar Georgetown Hospital looks much older than UCSF and the silver letters above the doors are off-center. We walk by a large framed photograph of Jackie Kennedy leaving the hospital with a baby. I'm not sure if the reverence for history is a good thing when it comes to neurosurgery, a discipline that has advanced to using lasers, but the atmosphere achieves professional and inviting.

Based on the website, Dr. Kevin McGrail sounds important. He's been the chair of neurosurgery for almost twenty years and I'm a little worried that my problems aren't important enough to warrant his time. After the fiasco with Dr. Carroll, I'm anxious that another doctor is going to judge me for a devolving medical condition that I don't fully understand. We're waiting at the elevator when he arrives behind us. Delightfully, he is carrying a donut.

"Dr. McGrail!" a hospital worker greets him. "How are things?"

He's pleasant, jovial even, and he waves to her as she pushes her cart down the hallway. I look at Chris. *This is our guy! With a donut!*

"Hi, Dr. McGrail," I venture. "We're about to have a meeting with you at nine thirty."

"Oh, is that right?" He holds the door for us as we all enter the elevator. I tell him that I'm coming from UCSF, from Dr. McDermott.

He's generous with his praise of both.

After I check in at the desk and complete paperwork, I join Chris in the waiting area. Soon we're called back to an exam room by Shannon, an energetic physician's assistant. We walk her through my story and then Dr. McGrail joins us in the room. Dr. McGrail is brisk and moves through conversation relatively quickly, sometimes interrupting to move things along, but he's entirely personable. Before looking at any film, he rolls his stool over and faces us.

How's your overall health otherwise? What kind of work do you do? Where did you go to school? And what do you do, sir? And how long have you been married? Any kids? Two boys! How old are the boys? Congratulations! And the surgery for the meningioma was after the kids?

He reviews the MRI images I've brought along on CDs.

"Cleaner than a hound's tooth!" he says. "This is great-looking post-op; he did a nice job here."

Dr. McGrail agrees that I can't drive until I'm stabilized on medication, which is frustrating but not unexpected. Next steps: Start an anti-seizure medication and schedule a follow-up appointment with Dr. Gholam Motamedi, the epilepsy neurosurgeon at Georgetown. We leave the hospital with smiles and high-fives for the entire team. This whole seizure thing was blown out of proportion. Right?

—

In the midst of all these doctor appointments, I take my bike in for a tune-up, redecorating it with bright pink grips and a new bike lock. A friend even sends me a little vase to hang on the handlebars. I'm doing the Jen thing again, distracting from the uncontrollable by reassuring everyone that I'm good, all good, who doesn't want a new biking hobby? *The tumor was benign!* I'm still out of the woods.

Soon after, Dr. Motamedi's office calls. Normally, he has a three-month waitlist, but apparently he's free at 3pm today. Can I make it? *Thanks, Bigness.* I cancel my meetings and take a Lyft over to Georgetown after lunch, picking up a lemon loaf on the way.

Dr. Motamedi is quiet and very smart, deliberate with his words. He smiles at the pastry and asks me many questions. I tell him about the Russian grandmother's voice during seizures.

"Do you have a Russian grandmother?" he asks.

"Nope."

"Is there someone else in your life *like* a Russian grandmother?"

"Nope."

"Are you sure she's Russian?"

"Nope."

"Interesting."

Dr. Motamedi takes no notes during our conversation. In a quick reverse move, he wants me to taper off the meds that Dr. McGrail just ordered me to start. Instead, he wants me to do an ambulatory EEG and he doesn't want anti-seizure medication to mess with that data. Between coaching sessions, I coordinate insurance and schedule the procedure.

On the day of the EEG, we drop the kids at Steve's and drive to Woodbridge, where an aide glues thirty-three electrodes across my head and chest, wrapping it all with gauze. I'm not allowed to take a shower for four days and must be within six feet of a video camera at all times. The camera will observe me working and mothering and cooking and sleeping. The goal is to capture a seizure on film.

When the aide finishes placing the electrodes, I peek in a mirror to see her work. Instantly, it's five years ago in ICU. My head is wrapped and there's no visible hair; Chris looks like he's seeing a ghost. The whole experience is familiar to us in the way it's unknown. In ten years of marriage, we've had too many of these appointments, meetings where we leave with strange instructions, follow-ups scheduled in bland office buildings that downplay how scared you might want to be.

I'm attached to this contraption on Noah's ninth birthday, which means that all family photos show a normal-looking family and me, Gauze Head. I wear large earrings and a bright dress to make up for it, but it's clear that I'm faking normalcy. In the mirror, I look sick. Maybe I am sick?

Where is The Bigness? I start pulling away from Chris and the kids. Instead of reading bedtime stories, I wipe down the kitchen counters and suggest that we watch TV to zone out after the kids are in bed.

Don't love me too much, I think. *If I die, I don't want you to be even sadder.*

I know grief is impossible to prevent. And yet.

~

Over four days, not one seizure is recorded. Dr. Motamedi uses this information to prescribe medication that will ramp up every two weeks until I'm at the full dose. These meds set a new rhythm to my days: 8am while I'm packing lunches and 8pm while the boys are brushing their teeth.

By the time I get to the six-week check-up, I'm mostly at peace with the medication but really itching to drive. Woo, bikes! But also woo, normal life! I haven't had a seizure in two months and I'm excited to move past this wrinkle in my story, to cite an extra dose of gratitude at Thanksgiving later this week.

Dr. James, a doctor-in-training, enters the exam room and I play with a plastic model of a brain while he asks his questions.

"What's your favorite thing about the brain?" I interrupt.

"That you can remove a lot of it, actually, and it still works."

"Wow, weird answer." We laugh. "You know, someone once told me people use only ten percent of our brains. When I heard that, I wanted to use eleven percent."

"Yikes, I think we might be at nuclear war if we all did that," he says.

"Or world peace," I counter. Dr. James winks and goes to find Dr. Motamedi.

When they come back together, Dr. Motamedi runs through some questions about side effects of the medications, reviews the EEG results, and starts winding down our conversation. Things are looking good, he says.

"Great," I say. "Well, before we get out of here, I have two things I want to check in on."

Dr. Motamedi nods.

"First, driving. How soon can that happen?"

I've been assuming that I'm an outlier, an exception to the Virginia DMV's rule. I've played nice with these doctors, I did their fancy EEG and took my meds like a good soldier. Not to mention, I haven't had loss of awareness in *any* of my seizures for five years. Surely now that I'm on medication, they'll let me drive.

"Six months."

"Sorry?"

"In six months you can email me the DMV form and I'll fill it out for you."

I'm speechless. *Six more months.* I do a mental calculation. Six months from now is *May.* May is almost summer. May is nearly the end of the school year. I'll end up relying on Chris and riding a fucking bike for almost the whole of my boys' first and third grades. Again, my body has failed me, changed what I thought my life would be. Again, I'm trapped.

"Okay . . . what about alcohol?"

Dr. Motamedi shakes his head.

"No alcohol?"

"Professionally, I need to tell you no alcohol. Alcohol on seizure medication is not recommended."

"Okay . . . for like, *the rest of my life?*"

He nods, reluctantly.

As we wrap up the appointment, I'm pleasant, even funny, with Dr. Motamedi and Dr. James, in the way we can move through surreal moments as plain old liars. My eyes tear up in the elevator as I head to the lab for bloodwork, but I hold it together while a nurse sticks me with a needle, even trading small talk about her holiday plans. Inside, my lying heart is so broken. The finish line has been moved once again.

It's Tuesday before Thanksgiving and it's rush hour, so, of course, there are no Lyfts and now I'm stuck at Georgetown Hospital, waiting. I follow a sign for the hospital chapel, find a pew, and cry. Housekeepers are cleaning the floor in the narthex and when they leave, I grant myself sobs, ugly stinging howls. My KN95 mask is snotty and soaked. Unlike the meditation room at UCSF, this chapel is full of biblical images and not a single aspect of it is comforting to me. I don't sense The Bigness in any of these decorations. Grief—what I believed to be healed but which may have just been sealed off—floods my body. I want my angel rep, I miss Dr. McDermott and UCSF, I didn't want this story to follow me. Now it's persisted across state lines.

People numb themselves to live through horrible news all the time; it's my turn. When I get home I tell Chris and the boys that I'm not good company and hole up in our bedroom, alone. As long as I'm watching an episode of a new TV drama, I can forget about my life, but when I take a break to get food, reality descends and I quickly start the next episode, repeatedly diving into forty-eight minutes of diversion. What's always unclear is how far I still have to fall. Maybe this is the bottom—but I don't know. I really just don't know.

Eight am take meds, 8pm take meds. You want your license back, Jen? Six months without a seizure. Go.

CHAPTER 31

THE THING ABOUT a benign brain tumor is that you think the craniotomy is the end of it. They take your face and skull apart, they put it back together, and then you recover. It's really very bad, but one day, a few years later, when stuck in traffic, you think, "Damn, now *that* was really something."

The thing about encountering God is that you think believing is the end of it. You felt a presence, you saw the visions, you took huge risks that affected the trajectory of your life. The math of these decisions only makes sense if God exists. Right?

Shortly after Christmas, Chris takes the boys to the bookstore and gives me a few hours alone. I can't drive, so I'm free to do what I want in the house: read, bake, knock out email, work on the book. Instead, I decide to elaborately call in the Divine.

I light a candle, successfully fumble the clasp on my sapphire necklace, and slip on the bright yellow socks from ICU.

I'm here, I say out loud. *Please tell me if I'll be okay.*

Silence.

The acappella recording of *Once in Royal David's City* is loud when I play it in the empty house; still, I wait for guidance.

Nothing.

Next, I play Avicii's song, *For a Better Day*. I skip through *The*

Beautiful Dream in my head, remembering the women, going home, necklaces made of light. I'm provoking a response, trying to trick the system back into the original glitch.

Still, nothing.

I sit in meditation, visualizing Plucky Institute. Those green fields, that building! I peek out of our bedroom window. *Was this what I saw? Was it not a piece of land, but a yard with a soccer goal and some garden boxes? Did I somehow mix things up?*

The candle melts and soon the kids will be home. Nothing's coming to save me this time. This is what I believe.

—

The reason I don't yet have a tattoo is that I haven't found anything that will always, eternally be true. I explain this to Steve over pizza one night.

"I probably encounter something once a week that makes me think oh, *that's* the tattoo I should get. But by the next week, it's somehow not as valid."

"Like what?"

"Like a song lyric or a famous quote or a symbol, I guess."

"What about Plucky's logo?"

I choke on my root beer.

"What am I, a piece of human swag? No, I'm saying if I have something *tattooed* on my body that I'm going to see every day and explain to people all the time, it has to be something I'll never get sick of. Something that is just so unshakable that it will be true until the day that I die."

Steve raises his eyebrows, takes a sip of his beer.

"That's a pretty high bar for a tattoo."

I never thought of it like that.

⌒

Aaron is having repeat nightmares about our cat dying and about losing us, his parents. I'm half asleep when I console him in the middle of the night, but the next morning I'm thinking about it as I pour his cereal.

"Hey buddy, I wanted to tell you something. You know how you've been having some bad dreams lately?"

He nods.

"Well, if you ever get scared or overwhelmed when you have a bad dream, you can always whisper, 'God be with me.' That's something I do if I'm really scared."

Aaron looks up, interested.

"Because God is always there, right?"

This is more direct than I've ever been with my six-year-old about The Bigness.

"Yeah, I think we're never alone and something big always loves us. That's what I believe."

Even as I say the words to him, I'm stretching the truth. The experiences of the past five years of my life have twisted and erased and complicated and evolved everything I knew before. *Where is God?* I lose her. *Here is God.* I find her.

Since brain surgery, I say three prayers every night after I turn off the light:

Thank you for this day.
Thank you for this life.
Thank you for this body.

I pause between each statement to rewind the day and find gratitude for a moment or two. I revisit my life and remember my story.

I take quick stock of my body and feel its weight on the mattress, as scarred and medicated as it now must be.

Thank you. Thank you. Thank you.

Sometimes at the grocery store I look at everyone's heads.

You have a brain in there, I think. *How is your brain?*

The older I get and the more people I encounter, this I understand: Everyone has something wrong. A lie, a break, a soft spot where it should be hard, a misfortune, a surprise, a weakness. Of course, there are many positive aspects to our lives, too. If not, how could we keep going? But no one escapes imperfection, and exploring our craters is where we find hope.

Health is not a binary. Faith is not a binary. *What else do I believe?*

I believe in being honest about my spirituality and in talking about things I can't understand. I believe that my family and friends may or may not believe the same, and that it's not my mission or job to change anyone's mind.

I believe in science and technology and math. I believe that many lives are saved every day because of humans' progress in these areas. I also believe that The Bigness may never be defined or proven in a laboratory.

I believe that life is what you make of it except when life makes it for you. Both options come with pressures and pearls.

I believe in coincidences, wild circumstances with incredible odds, even though I can never quite decipher what they're trying to tell me. I believe that some people have an easier time connecting to the unknown. Some of them might be called mediums.

I believe in tarot cards and journaling and asking yourself questions to figure out what you really want. I believe in coaching when you can't find your answers yourself. I believe that we all know, deep inside, who we want to be, and I believe that a worthy coach helps you hear it.

I believe in beloveds we lost too early and beloveds that are somehow, miraculously, still hanging on, waiting for an invisible permission slip to pass.

I believe that one day I will find out what happens when we die. I believe that the afterlife might be a fabulous brunch spent reconnecting with favorite people, an infinity of long conversations and coffee refills. I believe that you get a chance to come back and try it again, if you want.

At a minimum, I believe that the afterlife is more than nothing and that there's something giant out there. Because of this, I'm not afraid of death. One day I'll meet The Bigness and Grandma God and my angel rep and everything I've seen in dreams and I'll say, *Couldn't you have told me more?*

One day I'll know how it all works. Living this life and writing this book has made my own magic manifest. Today, as with most days, I believe in everything.

⌒

Before it gets too cold, I take my bike out for one last afternoon ride. I have a few hours before my next coaching call and, for once, I'm not using the time to run an errand or volunteer at the school. Instead, I'm following a new route that I've mapped out, something scenic. An old train line nearby was converted to a bike path. I'd like to explore it.

The first part of the ride is hard to memorize; I have to keep checking the map to confirm which streets to take. Even once I get to the bike path, I must cross a few busy roads, anticipate cars that could appear behind sharp turns, wait out some red lights. After a few intersections, I check the map again. No crossroads for now; looks like I've got a nice stretch ahead of me through the woods.

It's midday and the path isn't busy so I settle back onto my seat and take in my surroundings. The leaves are near the end of their cycles, soon to fall, but for now they're holding on. I hear birds, many of whom will be leaving soon for the winter. I sense the crackling of my new tires as they propel me forward. A dog barks, a bike bell rings. It's quiet in these woods. I'm glad to be here.

For now, on this path, I am well.

For now, on this path, I am safe.

For now, on this path, my ride is unfolding with ease.

And on this path, for as long as I am here, I am not alone.

This is what I believe.

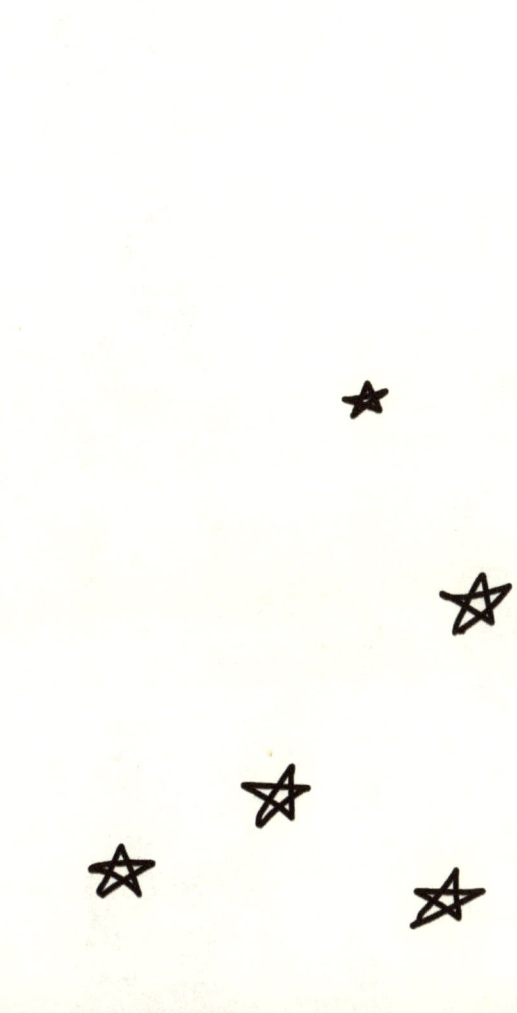

EPILOGUE

FOR ANYONE STRUGGLING to see possibility in their life this morning, and for anyone weighed down by burden or illness, especially . . .

I've added names to this list at church and I've watched some names move from this one to the next.

For all those we have lost, who we long to see again, especially . . .

After the intercessor reads the names, we're invited to add our own, out loud or in our hearts. This is when, anytime that I'm in a church, I quietly share Levi's name.

Levi Felix died on January 11, 2017, six months after I had coffee with him and Brooke, less than twelve months after his craniotomy. He was thirty-two.

Sometimes we're most changed by the people we hardly know, whose presences whisper past but thunder in their wake. Levi is more to me than someone I met two times. Levi represents what could have been, the tragedy of a cancerous brain tumor for someone in his early thirties, only starting his life. I say Levi's name because I got what he did not—a longer life to live. In honor of him, I try to stretch my life to maximum effect.

This doesn't mean that I don't feel down or get grumpy or resent others or take shortcuts, but, as often as possible, I do not forget the gift I've been given, and in the moments that invite my biggest self-doubts, I surrender to everything bigger than me.

Why me? I ask when I take new risks with Plucky.

Why me? I ask when my kids are thriving in their new school.

Why me? I ask when my MRI shows no tumor recurrence.

Why me? I ask when I doubt the validity of this entire book and my faith.

Levi Felix and his legacy and all The Bignesses from way beyond correct me.

Why NOT you, Jen?

Why not me? I wonder. So I step up and go on.

ACKNOWLEDGMENTS

THANK YOU, FIRST and foremost, to Chris, Noah, and Aaron. You are the main characters of my story, my beloved cheerleaders, and the reasons I'll always fight to live.

Indescribable gratitude to my medical team, including Dr. Michael McDermott, Jennifer Viner, Dr. Michael Safaee, Dr. Robert Darflinger, Dr. Tina T. Shih, the amazing nurses of UCSF Parnassus (especially Ron, Elisha, and Arma), and Dr. Kevin McGrail and Dr. Gholam Motamedi and their teams at Georgetown University Hospital.

An enormous thank you to my parents, siblings, and extended family members, whose love, support, texts, visits, care packages, and encouragement kept me going. Heartfelt thanks to the many folks who participated in our meal trains, donated through GoFundMe, gave cards or flowers or get-well gifts or hugs before and after surgery. Big love to dear friends who cheered me on during this long publishing process: my Muhlies, the Dragon girls book club, friends locally and abroad. Thanks to Reddit for Chris's generous caregiver leave.

More thanks to all members of my writing community: beta readers (Laura Mamelok, Rolph Blythe, Sarah Kersh, Emily Ford, Leigh Somerville, Ed Godbois, Shannon Duescher, Liz Tichenor,

Jeannie Koops, Eve Ettinger, Jess Farris), the Barrelhouse peeps and The Poets (Courtney Leblanc and Dan Brady), Book Buddies, Virginia Center for the Creative Arts, and Jane Vandenburgh and the Djerassi crew. Thanks to Jess Gould for being a copyediting doula, Matt Roeser for the cover magic, Zoe Norvell for designing the book guts.

Thank you to my Plucky community, including industry colleagues, SNYAM alumni, and coaching clients, whose abilities to find new perspectives and ways forward are incessantly inspiring. Thanks to Sheila Kenny for her calm and kind support. Thanks especially to Banfield, whose random "You're Jen Dary!" comment at a dinner party finally pushed me to get this book done.

Finally, to my spiritual crew and The Bigness, who drop acorns at my feet all day, every day: Thank you for my life. The abundance is overwhelming.

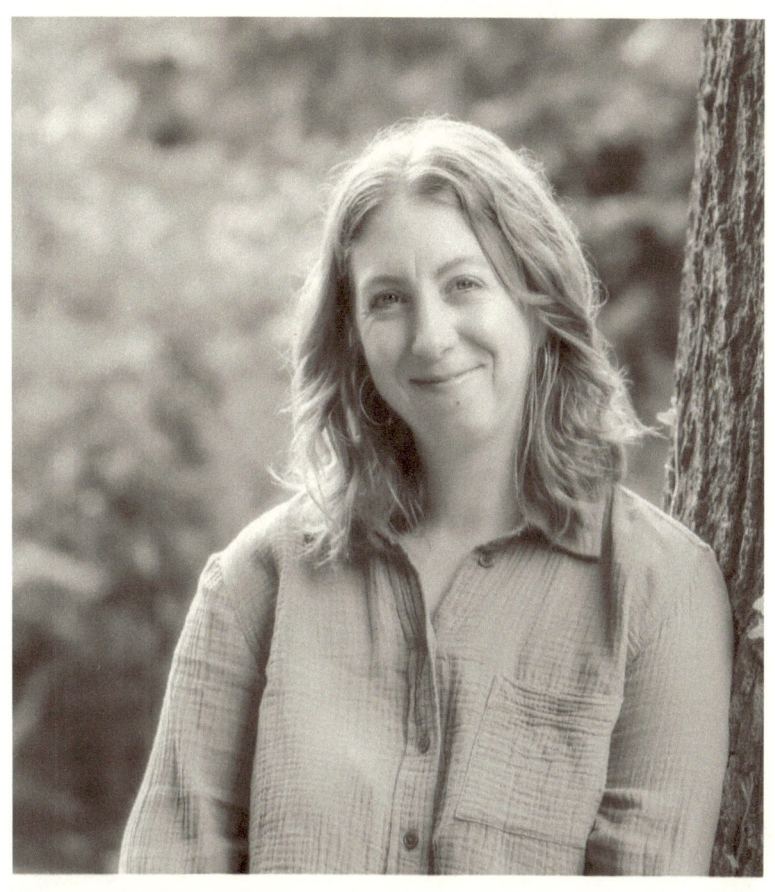

JEN DARY is a writer and leadership coach whose work explores the intersection of identity, belief, and personal transformation. She lives in Northern Virginia with her husband and sons. *I Believe in Everything* is her first book.

jendarywriter@gmail.com

@jendarywriter on Instagram